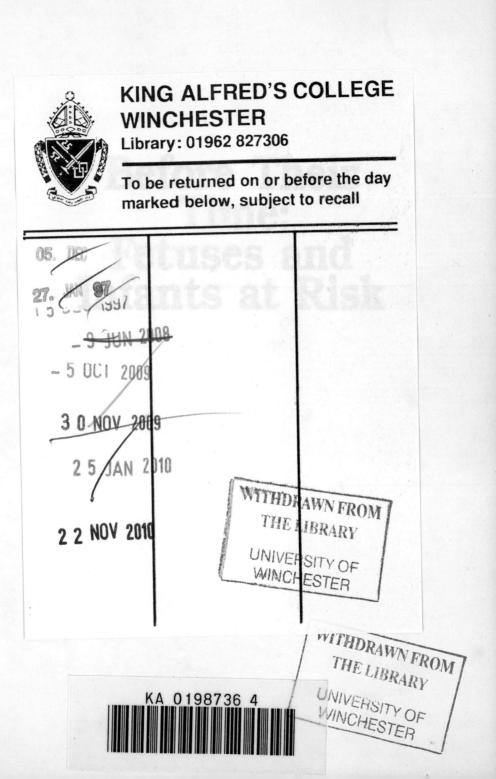

**Monographs of the
American Association
on Mental Retardation, 16**

Michael J. Begab, Series Editor

Before Their Time: Fetuses and Infants at Risk

by

Libby G. Cohen
University of Southern Maine

Published by
American Association on Mental Retardation
1719 Kalorama Road, NW
Washington, DC 20009

The points of view herein are those of the authors and do not necessarily represent the official policy or opinion of the American Association on Mental Retardation. Publication does not imply endorsement by the Editor, the Association, or its individual members.

No. 16, Monographs of the American Association on Mental Retardation (ISSN 0895-8009)

Library of Congress Cataloging-in-Publication Data is available.
CIP Card #90-14516

Printed in the United States of America

ISBN 0-940898-26-8

To Les and Seth

Table
of
Contents

Foreword

Before Their Time is a book for professionals and lay audiences. Libby Cohen is an educator who became interested and concerned primarily with fetal and neonatal risk factors. She observed the impact of medical controversies on society, professionals and concerned parents and families seeking care and advice. The decision to do such a book did not come easily. The outcome provides reassurance to her and all who might otherwise hesitate to speak out on ethical issues that relate directly to their work and their lives.

The book warns of complex problems that lie ahead, with the startling advantages that new technology will bring. The greatest contribution of the book is to peel away the obfuscation that covers the ethical controversies with which society must come to grips. Although medical ethics is an old and sophisticated field, current issues have risen to the top of the national agenda, i.e., right to life, right to choose, neonatal intensive care, organ and tissue waiting lists (who gets on and whose organs can be donated), informed consent, and legal death.

These and other urgent issues might not have been projected so precipitously into the forefront of the nation's conscience if technology had not emerged so suddenly. For instance, because we know many additional facts about the emerging fetus, information can be added to case conferences involving parents. The issues of motherhood and fatherhood have been drawn into a vast arena they share with attendant physicians, medical ethicists, legal scholars (on the left and the right), legislators, and family policy advisors.

Throughout the book, Dr. Cohen shows an intent to inform, but not to persuade. This is not an advocacy book. Although advocacy provides a much-needed source of strength in human service fields, if introduced between the lines in a scholarly book, it clouds the issues. Dr. Cohen understands this and, consequently, seeks primarily to inform. Her information is appropriately comprehensive and interpretative; but the interpretation sections point the way to further sources and to additional interpretations, and do not attempt to persuade the reader to accept a predetermined point of view.

Instead, she points out directions for study and further research. This approach provides reassurance for those of us who although greatly interested and concerned, may at times feel constrained by the doctrinaire statements of protagonists and the hurried language of reporters.

Some may not wish to wait for the processes of scholarship and the measured pace of ethical analysis, but all of us must "seek wisdom in the use of our human made tools. . .We must always be keenly aware of our inescapable frailties. . ." (p.301) and the possible failure of our vision. Public policy develops out of the interaction between ethical beliefs and technological progress.

The pace of this interaction is accelerating. It's as though new issues of morality are thrust upon us with each new edition of the daily paper or weekly news magazine. Each year, new living conditions are shaped by legal decisions and health care is replanned along lines determined by legislative, economic and social forces. Special advocacy groups vie with each other in influencing public policy.

It appears that the mechanisms and the soul of our democratic society are being tested. For each of us the implied obligations are many. We should, as a bare minimum, seek to be well informed about the advances and the dangers that technologies hold forth for our future. This is a book to be read and discussed. Send a copy to a friend.

Richard Schiefelbusch
University of Kansas

Preface

Each year, thousands of newborns who are critically ill are admitted to neonatal intensive care units. These infants, many of whom will survive, are kept alive through the use of sophisticated technologies and highly trained medical personnel. Entering a neonatal intensive care unit, the visitor is struck by the bright lights, which shine day and night, the whirring machines, the blinking monitors, and tiny infants who are connected to respirators and catheters. Some of these infants have disabilities or will develop them; they have barely begun life. It is "before their time."

We are also faced with other dilemmas. Advances in technology have given us the ability to identify many disorders *in utero*. Some fetuses can now be treated *in utero*; for others treatments have not yet been discovered. What are the dilemmas that are faced when a fetus is identified as having a potential disability?

This book discusses some of the ethical dilemmas that are raised when fetuses and infants are identified as having disabilities or potential disabilities. Rapid developments in medical technology have far outpaced the establishment of ethical and legal standards in this area. It has been through case law rather than statutory law, with the exception of the homocide and feticide laws, that some protection has been granted to the infant and the fetus.

I have tried to present a balanced approach to this potentially inflammatory topic. There are limitations. While I have reviewed much of the literature, I realize that I have made omissions. Even as I write, there are new discoveries in medical technology. In the political arena, many of these issues are hotly debated.

A note on the terminology. "Disabled" does seem to be a very appropriate adjective to use when describing children and adults. But using the word "disabled" to refer to a fetus with a severe medical condition may offend some readers. Thus, I have decided to refer to fetuses as "having conditions that are disabling or potentially disabling."

As used in this book, the term "severely disabled" does *not* refer to the psychometric use of the term as defined by AAMR. Rather, it refers to infants who are critically ill and who have life threatening conditions; some have severe cognitive disabilities. Many of them are born prematurely because of inadequate prenatal care or because their mothers abused drugs and/or alcohol. Some of the infants born with congenital disorders such as microcephaly,

Down syndrome, and spina bifida also have medical conditions that jeopardize their survival.

I am very grateful for the gentle encouragement and kind words of the editor, Michael Begab. My sincere thanks are extended to the two Rebeccas: Rebecca Neidetcher and Rebecca Smith—and to Carrie Beaulieu for their assistance with library research. Their help and dedication are very much appreciated. I am grateful to Loraine Spenciner for her insightful comments.

My deep gratitude is extended to the librarians at the University of Southern Maine, Jim Brady, Casandra Fitzherbert, Rose Hickey, Phyllis Locke, Sheila Johnson, and especially to Franklin Talbot. Pearl Wuthrich provided valuable secretarial assistance.

I am grateful to the University of Southern Maine for granting me a sabbatical to complete this project. Finally, my family, Les and Seth, provided encouragement and support far beyond what I deserve.

The Fetus with a Disability or Potential Disability

Chapter 1

With rapid advances in prenatal diagnostic techniques, many fetuses who are identified as having a disability or potential disability would not have been identified several years ago. Fetuses that have been injured because of actions that occurred prior to conception, during gestation, during unsuccessful abortions, or during birth are fetuses that are disabled or potentially disabled. Fetuses are especially vulnerable because they may be singled out for special treatment (*e.g.*, abortion, less than vigorous medical intervention) because they have a disability or a potential disability.

This chapter will examine the legal issues that have been raised when a fetus that is disabled or potentially disabled is identified. This discussion will document the development of the emerging rights of the fetus, will highlight some of the dilemmas that exist, and will identify areas that need resolution and further study. Almost all of the legal issues that will be discussed involve case law rather than statutory law, because it has been through court decisions, with the exception of the homicide and feticide laws, that some protection has been granted to the fetus. The issues are complex; the needs of women, men, families, children, and the fetus must be considered. It is hoped that an examination of these issues will contribute to an understanding of them and to their resolution.

THE BEGINNING OF RIGHTS

In 1884, the Supreme Judicial Court of Massachusetts handed down a landmark decision regarding the relationship between a mother and her fetus. In an opinion written by Justice Oliver Wendall Holmes, the Massachusetts Supreme Court, in the case *Dietrich v. Inhabitants of Northhampton* (1884), denied that a mother could seek damages for her fetus that miscarried when she fell on an unrepaired road. Justice Holmes ruled that the fetus was part of the mother when the accident occurred and was not a separate entity at the time of the accident.

The *Dietrich* case was precedent setting because it was the first time in which recovery for damages incurred by a fetus was considered. This case remained a precedent for 62 years, until 1946, when a ruling in *Bonbrest v. Kotz* (1946), reversed the *Dietrich* decision and ruled that a doctor was responsible for injuries to a fetus during delivery (Collins, 1983-84; Osborne, 1984).

1

The *Bonbrest* decision was a precedent-setting ruling because it recognized that a child could recover for injuries incurred while still a fetus (Osborne, 1984). This case alleged that a physician had acted improperly during delivery and that the child had been injured during birth. The *Bonbrest* decision held, that, if a child were born alive, then the child could bring a case before the courts and could recover damages for injuries incurred while s/he was a fetus. (Osborne, 1984). This case was important because, for the first time, viability was emphasized as the determining factor in awarding damages. As of this writing, the majority of states have rejected the *Dietrich* ruling and rely on the *Bonbrest* ruling (Beal, 1984).

Many courts since *Bonbrest* have used the standard of viability as a basis for granting or denying an award of damages involving the negligent injury of a fetus. The point at which viability is determined is one of the central issues in a discussion of legal protection of the fetus. With advances in medicine, fetuses that were once thought not to be viable do survive.

Many judicial decisions use the term "viable" and interpret this as the point at which the fetus is able to survive, even with artificial means, outside of the mother. U.S. Supreme Court Justice Harry Blackmun, who wrote the majority opinion in 1973 for the *Roe v. Wade* (1973) decision, defined fetal viability as the point at which the fetus is capable of meaningful life outside the uterus.

The general consensus is that viability does not occur until after 28 weeks of gestation, but medical advances have challenged this belief. Viability testing is inexact at best, and it is highly unlikely that any fetuses can be kept alive outside the mother prior to 22 weeks of gestation. Because of this, the courts have been criticized for using viability as a legal standard in deciding the merits of a case.

In *Kelly v. Gregory* (1953), the New York Supreme Court Appellate Division decision granted recovery for prenatal injuries that were incurred any time after conception. Today, it is well accepted that a child who is born alive can recover for prenatal injuries that were incurred before or after viability (Osborne, 1984). Osborne summarized the application of this ruling:

> Today, of the thirty-six jurisdictions which allow a cause of action for prenatal torts, seventeen do not require a child to be viable at the time of its injury in order to recover. Nineteen jurisdictions retain the viability standard, but eleven of these used the standard in cases which involved a stillborn fetus. Three cases involve a child who died shortly after live birth. There are fourteen jurisdictions which have not ruled on the scope of prenatal tort liability. Given recent trends, it appears that in time all jurisdictions will grant a cause of action to a child who is injured between its conception and birth by the wrongful conduct of another (Osborne, 1984, pp.681-682).

PRECONCEPTION TORTS

In the chronology of court cases concerning the fetus, there are several cases that have addressed the rights of a fetus even before conception has occurred. These cases are known as preconception torts (Andrews, 1984). Several courts have ruled that a child can bring an action before the courts for events that occurred even before the child was conceived; several other cases have reached opposing opinions.

Piper v. Hoard (1887) was the first case that considered damages for a negligent act that occurred prior to conception. A child's mother was involved in a land fraud scheme before the child was conceived, and the child sought damages for negligence. A New York court awarded damages but did not address the issue that the child had not even been conceived when the fraud had occurred. The court based its decision on the belief that the mother would eventually give birth to a child anyway (Andrews, 1984).

Jorgenson v. Meade Johnson Laboratories (1972), was brought on behalf of twins with Down syndrome. The mother had taken oral contraceptives that were alleged to have caused chromosomal deformities. Although the case was dismissed by a lower court, a higher court in voiding the lower court's ruling seemed to recognize the existence of a cause for preconception injuries (Andrews, 1984) and the rights of the child before conception. Another case, *Renslow v. Mennonite Hospital* (1977), awarded damages to a child with a disability who was born nine years after the mother had received improper blood transfusions.

Not all preconception torts have awarded damages for injuries that occurred prior to conception (Andrews, 1984). In *Albala v. City of New York* (1981), the New York Supreme Court heard a case concerning a woman who, during an abortion, had her uterus damaged. Subsequently, she became pregnant and gave birth to a child who was brain damaged, allegedly because of the damage to the uterus.

In this case, the court denied the cause for action because, if the court had granted recovery for damages it would have the undesirable impact of encouraging the practice of "defensive medicine":

> A physician faced with the alternative of saving a patient's life by administering a treatment involving the possibility of adverse consequences to later conceived offspring of the patient would, if exposed to liability of the magnitude considered in this case, undoubtedly be inclined to advise against the treatment rather than risk the possibility of having to recompense a child born with a handicap. Accordingly, society as a whole would bear the cost of our placing physicians in direct conflict between their moral duty to patients and the proposed legal duty to those hypothetical future generations outside the immediate zone of danger (*Albala v. City of New York* (1981), pp.788-789).

McAuley v. Wills (1983) was another case in which recovery for a preconception tort was denied (Andrews, 1984). In this case, a woman was injured in a car accident. The following year she gave birth to a child who died the day after birth because of problems during the birth process that were attributable to the mother's injuries. This was a precedent-setting case because the court's ruling distinguished between the mother's injuries and the intervening negligence of the doctor:

> While denying liability for a preconception tort, this decision is a useful precedent due to its analysis of the duty, foreseeability, and proximate cause issues. The court acknowledged that a preconception tort is compensable in certain situations, but recognized the intervening negligence of the delivering physician as the proximate cause of the injury (Andrews, 1984, p.92).

A review of preconception cases shows that the courts have been inconsistent in awarding damages. While the early cases *Piper v. Hoard* (1887), *Jorgenson v. Meade Johnson Laboratories* (1972), and *Renslow v. Mennonite Hospital* (1977) recognized a basis for preconception torts, later cases such as *Albala v. City of New York* (1981) and *McAuley v. Wills* (1983), seem to have reversed the reasoning of the earlier cases. This is an area of the law that will require much more clarification. Perhaps the legal basis for preconception torts does not lie with the courts. This may be a statutory area and it should probably be left to the state legislatures to define the legal conditions for preconception torts.

However, state legislatures have been reluctant to enact laws relating to preconception because many other sensitive issues will be involved. The rights of the mother will be juxtaposed with the rights of the fetus; the issues of whether the fetus is a person and when the fetus attains personhood will be raised; the responsibilities of physicians prior to conception will have to be examined; and the regulation of birth control will be debated. Because of the sensitivity of these and other issues, the area of preconception torts will remain unclear and the rights of the fetus, in this area, will remain undefined.

WRONGFUL BIRTH, WRONGFUL LIFE, AND WRONGFUL DEATH

Protection of the fetus, particularly with respect to the right to recover damages when there has been some negligence toward the fetus after conception, has received attention by the courts. Negligence cases can be divided into three categories: wrongful birth, wrongful life, and wrongful death. Wrongful birth cases involve claims by some parents that their child should never have been born. Wrongful birth suits are brought by parents who allege that medical personnel have, through negligence, denied parents the opportunity for an abortion (Steinbock, 1986). Parents ask for relief from the mental, financial, and physical suffering of having and raising a handicapped child.

Wrongful life cases claim that the child's life is worse than death or nonexistence (Parness & Pritchard, 1982). Wrongful death cases claim that the child should not have died and that were it not for certain circumstances, the child could have survived. Currently, all states have wrongful death statutes for persons who died because of some wrongful act. Table 1.1 provides a summary of the landmark decisions in these areas.

TABLE 1.1

Preconception Torts, Wrongful Birth, Wrongful Life, Wrongful Death Landmark Cases (U. S.)

Preconception Torts

Case	Year	Ruling
Piper v. Hoard (New York)	1887	Awarded damages for a negligent act that occurred prior to conception
Jorgenson v. Meade Johnson Laboratories (Oklahoma)	1973	Awarded damages to twins with Down Syndrome whose mother had taken birth control pills
Renslow v. Mennonite Hospital (Illinois)	1977	Awarded damages to a handicapped child born 9 years after the mother had received a blood transfusion
Albala v. City of New York (New York)	1981	Court denied claims by a woman who gave birth to a child who was brain damaged during birth because her uterus had been perforated in an abortion
McCauley v. Wills (Georgia)	1983	Court denied claims to a woman whose child died shortly after birth because of injuries she had sustained in an auto accident prior to conception

Wrongful Birth

Case	Year	Ruling
Bonbrest v. Kotz (Federal Circuit Court)	1946	Held a doctor responsible for injuries to a fetus during delivery
Kelly v. Gregory (New York)	1953	Court granted recovery for prenatal injuries that occurred anytime after conception
Jacob v. Theimer (Texas)	1975	Court awarded damages to a child whose mother had undiagnosed rubella

Wrongful Life

Case	Year	Ruling
Zepeda v. Zepeda (Illinois)	1963	Child brought suit against unmarried father because the child had been born a "bastard"

(continued on next page)

TABLE 1.1 *(continued)*

**Preconception Torts, Wrongful Birth, Wrongful Life, Wrongful Death
Landmark Cases (U. S.)**

Wrongful Life *(continued)*

Gleitman v. Cosgrove (New Jersey)	1967	Denied claims to a woman who alleged that a doctor had not informed her about the injuries that rubella can cause and she was unable to have an abortion
Curlender v. Bio-Science Laboratories (California)	1980	Court awarded damages because genetic screening tests for Tay-Sachs disease had been improperly analyzed and their child was born with this disease
Turpin v. Sortini (California)	1982	Court rejected the claims of a woman that her doctor had not informed her that it was possible that her child could be born deaf

Wrongful Death

Dietrich v. Inhabitants of Northhampton (Massachusetts)	1884	Denied claims to a woman who miscarried when she fell on an unrepaired road
Verkennes v. Corniea (Minnesota)	1949	First case to allow a wrongful death claim for a viable fetus that did not survive delivery
Endresz v. Friedberg (New York)	1969	Court denied claims to parents of twins who were stillborn after a car accident
Dunn v. Rose Way Inc. (Iowa)	1983	Court awarded damages to a father whose wife, child, and unborn child were killed in a car accident
Commonwealth v. Cass (Massachusetts)	1984	Massachusetts Supreme Court ruled that a viable fetus is a person

The viability of the fetus at the time of the action remains the standard that courts use to determine whether a wrongful act has occurred. Many states permit civil actions on behalf of a fetus when a fetus dies as the result of a negligent act (Osborne, 1984). While it is accepted that recovery for damages to a child that were incurred before or after viability can be sought, there is disagreement over whether recovery can be sought for damages to a fetus that is not viable.

Wrongful Birth

The courts have recognized that infants born alive who suffered some harm during gestation are entitled to some compensation. These claims have been brought on the grounds of "wrongful birth." In *Jacob v. Theimer* (1975), the court awarded damages to a child whose mother had rubella during pregnancy that was not diagnosed during the pregnancy. The court held that the mother's physician was responsible for past and future expenses of the child.

Wrongful Life

The term "wrongful life" first occurred in the case *Zepeda v. Zepeda* (1963), when a child whose parents had not married brought suit against his father because he had been born illegitimate (Stoutamire, 1981). The court dismissed the case because it felt it would be opening the door to additional cases. *Gleitman v. Cosgrove* (1967) was an important case in the chronology of wrongful life cases because the court denied the claims of wrongful life. The parents claimed that the physician had not informed the parents about the injuries that rubella can cause and, thus, the mother was unable to have an abortion.

In a case brought before the California Supreme Court, *Turpin v. Sortini* (1982), the parents alleged that they had not been informed that it was possible that their child could be born deaf. The court rejected their claims.

In *Curlender v. Bio-Science Laboratories* (1980), parents alleged that their child was born with Tay-Sachs disease because genetic tests had been improperly analyzed. In this case, the court recognized the wrongful life claims. The decision was that the infant, who brought the case along with the parents, was conceived because of improper genetic counseling. In deciding for the plaintiffs, the court interpreted the plaintiffs' claims for pain and suffering as being due to medical malpractice.

From 1963, with the *Zepeda* decision, to 1980, with the *Curlender* decision, the change in how the courts have viewed wrongful life cases has been enormous. The *Curlender* decision has highlighted moral and legal questions about society's treatment of persons who are disabled (Steinbock, 1986; Stoutamire, 1981).

How does a court go about deciding the amount of damages to compensate parents when they have a child who is severely disabled? What value does society place on the lives of children who may be completely dependent for the rest of their lives versus children who will be contributing members of society? Do we view children only for their economic value? If a fetus with a severe disability is diagnosed *in utero,* to what extent are parents obligated to abort the fetus for the good of society? Should only medical expenses be reimbursed? Should there be compensation for pain and suffering? Because the courts have found it difficult to quantify the monetary loss of an unborn child, they have vacillated in the amount and types of awards that have been made. The question of what types of awards should be made and the criteria on which to base these awards remains inconsistent:

Despite the concern of the courts with the issues of speculation and double recovery, parents have been able to recover for the wrongful death of their unborn child. Examples of elements of damages recoverable include the parents' out-of-pocket medical expenses, funeral expenses, and also the net value to the parents of the child's prospective services. Furthermore, it has been held that element of nonpecuniary loss, such as loss of society and companionship, may be recoverable (Osborne, 1984, pp.1677-1678).

Only three states—New Jersey, California, and Washington—have recognized wrongful life suits and three states—Minnesota, South Dakota, and Utah—have voted to prohibit them (Steinbock, 1986).

Wrongful Death

In 1949, the Minnesota Supreme Court in *Verkennes v. Corniea* was the first court to allow a wrongful death claim. Both the fetus and the mother did not survive the delivery and the father claimed that the deaths were caused by the negligence of the attending physician (Osborne, 1984).

In another case, *Endresz v. Friedberg* (1969), as a result of a car accident, a woman who was seven months pregnant was injured and gave birth to stillborn twins. The court ruled that damages could not be recovered by the parents.

In *Dunn v. Rose Way, Inc.* (1983), a mother, child, and an unborn child were killed in an accident with a trailer truck. The husband and father brought a suit on behalf of his wife, daughter, and unborn child. In an appeal, the Iowa Supreme Court ruled that damages could be granted because the father had lost the companionship, company, and services of the unborn child. The *Dunn* case recognized that parents could be compensated for the loss of an unborn child because of negligence.

In a seeming reversal of awarding damages for preconception torts, a 1984 Massachusetts Supreme Court (*Commonwealth v. Cass*) ruled, in a landmark decision, that a viable fetus is a person. A woman, eight and one-half months pregnant, was hit by a car. The fetus was delivered by Cesarean section but died because of injuries incurred in the accident. The court ruled that the decision granting the personhood of a fetus would not be applied in this case but in future cases.

A review of the preceding cases reveals the inconsistency of court decisions involving postconception torts. The courts have also vacillated in awarding damages in postconception cases. Andrews (1983-84) wrote that courts are uncertain about the limits of liability. Collins (1984) stated that liability depends on the time, the place, and the events surrounding the injury or death of the fetus. As a result of this inconsistency, prenatal rights and protections have not been clearly defined.

FETICIDE

While every state has laws that prohibit homicide, the extent to which these laws are applied to the termination of a fetus varies. Some states have specific laws that prohibit the intentional killing of a fetus; other states apply the homicide statutes in cases where the fetus is determined to have been viable.

In cases where the fetus could not have been born alive, the courts have not defined feticide as a crime (Goichman & Hirsh, 1984). Moreover, states vary in the types of punishments meted out to perpetrators of feticide. Many laws that seem to protect the fetus are actually designed to protect the mother (Parness, 1985).

In *Keeler v. Superior Court* (1970), the court found that a fetus was not a human being. Robert Keeler, divorced from his wife Teresa in September 1968, assaulted her when he discovered that she was pregnant by another man. Saying, "I'm going to stomp it out of you" (Webb, 1971, p.171), he killed the fetus. Although the age of the fetus was unclear, the evidence showed that it would have survived if it had been born alive (Webb, 1971). It seems that the courts will not convict a defendant of feticide unless the fetus is viable at the time of the criminal act and unless laws are specifically enacted that proscribe feticide (Goichman & Hirsh, 1984).

The criminal abortion laws are a specific set of laws designed to protect the fetus. Court decisions in criminal cases have generally treated cases involving the killing of a fetus more leniently than cases that considered the murder of infants. Several cases (*California v. Smith*, 1976; *Keeler v. Superior Court*, 1970; *Louisiana v. Brown*, 1979) ruled that a fetus, stillborn because of an attack on the mother, was not a person. Again, the viability of the fetus at the time of the assault was the central concern of the court.

ABORTION AND LIVE BIRTH

Nowhere do the rights of the fetus, the mother, and the newborn collide more abruptly than when an abortion the mother has arranged results in a live birth. Medical technology has made enormous strides; now, even very tiny newborns may survive independent of the mother. An infant born of a late abortion not only carries the risks associated with prematurity, but, in addition to not being wanted, may also have been damaged by the attempted abortion.

Mothers who have struggled with the decision of whether or not to carry to term a fetus diagnosed as having a handicap or a potential handicap (*e.g.*, Down syndrome, anencephaly, Tay-Sachs disease) may face other, more agonizing decisions about whether to permit treatment of the newborn or whether the treatment is in the best interests of the newborn (Rhoden, 1984).

Although several states have passed laws that in effect terminate parental rights when a late abortion results in a live birth, federal courts have ruled these laws to be unconstitutional (Rhoden, 1984). These rulings have had several implications for the rights of women. First, legalized abortion does not end a woman's right to custody of the child, if born alive. Second, women must be considered when treatment decisions are made about the child.

The occurrence of a live birth following a late abortion can be an agonizing situation for parents and for medical personnel whose training tells them that they should preserve life. But when the intended abortus is a fetus that has been diagnosed as having a disability or a potential disability, the dilemma becomes more acute. Hospitals and physicians are led to believe, through training and societal attitudes, that when a mother of a fetus with a disability or potential disability elects to have an abortion, that the desired outcome is the termination of the fetus, or feticide.

Many abortion decisions, based on the presence of a disabling condition, are not made until the second trimester because of the limitations of prenatal screening procedures. But, Collins (as quoted in Rhoden, 1984) has written that doctors may not be as aggressive in their treatment of newborns with disabilities that have survived an abortion:

> Where parents and doctor have agreed that because of genetic defects an abortion is medically prudent, physicians state they seldom, if ever, will violate parental wishes by attempting to resuscitate an abortus or by performing lifesaving procedures (Rhoden, 1984, p.1487).

Because so few handicapping or potentially handicapping conditions can be treated before or after birth, Rhoden (1984) has written that abortion remains the "treatment of choice" (p.1486). A woman, because she has chosen abortion:

> may desire feticide more explicitly and more strongly than is typical in ordinary elective abortion. In this situation she wants a baby but does not want this baby. She may believe this infant would suffer dreadfully or would lead such a limited existence that it should not be brought into the world. A physician who has performed amniocentesis and recommended abortion likewise may share these beliefs, and therefore, may feel even less inclined to resuscitate such an infant than one born alive from a regular abortion (Rhoden, 1984, p.1487).

PREVENTING BIRTH

Parness and Pritchard (1982) wrote that there are few laws that prevent birth. Almost every state at one time had involuntary sterilization laws. These were designed to prohibit the conception of persons who might be disabled or socially undesirable. The criminal incest laws were another set of laws that were intended to prevent birth and designed to protect the "well-being of persons not presently conceived" (Parness & Pritchard, 1982, p.289).

PROTECTION OF THE FETUS

Although the courts have refused to expand the homicide laws to include feticide, the Civil Rights Act provides that a viable fetus is a person (Goichman & Hirsh, 1984). Fetuses that are not yet viable remain in never-never land, caught between conflicting rights of the parents and societal attitudes and beliefs.

There have been several instances in which direct attempts have been made to protect a fetus. Many states do not have legal provisions for protecting a fetus. One major reason is that direct intervention means that if the fetus is taken into custody the mother must also be taken into custody.

Generally, the mother's rights have outweighed any the fetus may have. In the case *Jefferson v. Griffin Spalding County Hospital Authority* (1981), the Superior Court of Butts County, GA, ruled that a pregnant woman had to have a sonogram and a Cesarean section in order to protect the life of her unborn child. The mother had refused to undergo surgery and any blood transfusions, if needed, because of her religious beliefs. Because the fetus was viable, the court ruled that the state could take custody of the fetus (and the mother) (Manner, 1982; Parness & Pritchard, 1982).

Fetuses have been protected in other instances. A California woman who was 22 weeks pregnant suffered a seizure. She was pronounced "brain dead" and was kept alive for nine weeks until her child could be delivered. After the child was born, the mother was declared legally dead and life support was discontinued ("Life from Death," 1983).

In a 1986 case, a brain-dead woman who was pregnant with a 21-week-old fetus was the focus of a court case when her husband and another man, the father of the fetus, argued whether she should be maintained on life support equipment until the fetus was old enough to be viable. In this case, a Georgia court granted the father's request to keep the woman alive until the fetus could survive outside the mother ("Ruling by a Court Keeps Fetus Alive," 1986).

While there seems to be some legal protection for women, little consideration has been given to active protection of the fetus. Although Title VII of the Civil Rights Act bans sex discrimination during employment, there is a question as to whether this applies to women who are of childbearing age. In addition, the Federal Pregnancy Discrimination Act, which provides that pregnant employees must receive the same benefits as all other employees, may afford some protection (Lewin, 1988). Lewin (1988) also suggested that the solution may be to work toward making all workplaces safe; if certain substances are harmful to fetuses they may be harmful to adults, as well.

In addition, Lewin (1988) discussed the ethical and legal dilemmas posed when women of childbearing age and pregnant women work under conditions that are hazardous or potentially hazardous to the health of a fetus. Several research studies have shown that certain work conditions are associated with higher rates of miscarriage. Women who worked in rooms where computer chips are made and women who worked on video display terminals had high incidences of miscarriage.

Some women have asked for transfers because the conditions under which they work may be hazardous to a developing fetus. Employers nervous about liability suits have prevented women from working in jobs that may be dangerous to a developing fetus. Excluding women from certain working conditions may result in women not being hired for certain types of jobs. Some women see this protective exclusion as a form of sex discrimination:

> The legal status of protective exclusion remains unclear. Employers say they have to keep women out of dangerous jobs to avoid liability for miscarriage, birth defects, and other child bearing problems. But many women see the policies as a form of sex discrimination that unfairly treats all women as potential breeders and makes them less attractive job candidates (Lewin, 1988, p.A15).

Most of the child abuse and neglect laws do not include provisions for protection of the fetus (Parness, 1985). Recent concerns about the effect of unhealthy conditions in the workplace and in the environment on women, the addiction of fetuses on drugs, and the potential of abuse and neglect of infants once they are born has prompted some courts, environmental groups, and agencies to take actions to protect fetuses as well as those that have not yet been conceived.

In one case (Feron, 1988), a pregnant woman who had abused or neglected seven children was ordered by a judge to give up her baby at birth. This case also illustrated the conflicting attitudes society has toward the protection of the fetus. The judge claimed that, because the mother had such a record of abuse, it was up to her to prove that she could care for the infant. But, civil libertarians argued that the judge, by his actions, was according the fetus the rights of a person, and that this was improper.

The ethical and moral aspects of the issue of protection of the fetus have received considerable attention. Some of the questions that have been addressed include: At what point in its nine-month development does a fetus attain the status of a person? How do the state and society balance the rights of the mother with the emerging rights of the fetus? Do fetuses that are disabled or have the potential of being disabled require special legal considerations?

THE *ROE* DECISION

Any rights that the fetus might have are nullified when the mother has an abortion. The U. S. Supreme Court, on January 22, 1973, handed down two landmark decisions on abortion. In *Roe v. Wade* (1973), the majority opinion held that the decision to have an abortion was to be left to the woman and her doctor. In *Doe v. Bolton* (1973), the court ruled that permission by abortion committees and residency requirements were unnecessary. In a discussion of fetuses that are disabled or are potentially disabled, an examination of the *Roe* decision is critical. The U. S. Supreme Court ruled in the *Roe* case that the fetus was not a person and thus not protected under the 14th Amendment of the U. S. Constitution until it was viable. Only at the point of viability could the government regulate abortions in order to protect the life of the fetus (Cohen, 1986).

Kader (1980) has analyzed judicial decisions since the *Roe* decision and he has written that *Roe* has been interpreted in three different ways with regard to wrongful death cases:

> First, in an attempt to *deny recovery,* the courts have used *Roe* to support the argument that there should be no recovery because the fetus is not a "person" within the Fourteenth Amendment. Second, in an effort to *limit recovery* to viable fetuses, the decision has been used to support the argument that recovery should be allowed only when the fetus is viable because that is when the state's interest in prenatal life becomes "compelling" according to *Roe*. Finally, in an effort to *expand recovery,* the decision has been used to support the argument that recovery should be allowed because according to *Roe* the state does have an interest in prenatal life (Kader, 1980, p.663).

Thus, for fetuses that are disabled or have the potential of being disabled, if they are previable, selective abortions can be performed. For fetuses that are viable but sustain an injury and do not survive, wrongful death actions can be undertaken. For fetuses that are handicapped or have the potential of being handicapped and are viable, there seems to be some protection under the *Roe* decision. For injuries that have been caused by actions prior to conception, it is uncertain whether court actions can be successfully resolved.

The *Roe* decision has had a profound impact on society. While there continues to be intense controversy among persons favoring abortion, persons opposing abortion, and others who promote the rights of women, each year there has been an increase in the number of abortions that are performed in the United States. It is difficult to know how many of these abortions are performed because the fetus has been diagnosed as having a birth disorder. But with the increased ability to diagnose the presence of birth disorders early in the pregnancy, and with lowered medical risks associated with an abortion, it is apparent that some abortions are performed because a birth disorder has been diagnosed in the fetus.

The determination of viability is dependent upon a number of different factors: weight, health, and genetic characteristics of the fetus; health of the mother; and the quality of the prenatal care. Thus, a fetus carried by a woman with poor prenatal care and poor health may not be viable, while a fetus carried by a woman who has received adequate prenatal care and who is in good health may be viable (Scofield, 1982). Scofield (1982) has written that not only is viability a poor standard to use when deciding compensation to parents in wrongful death cases, but it also "raises serious constitutional equal protection issues" (1982, p.807).

Further, Parness (1985) suggested that the *Roe* decision implicitly held that the fetus should receive some respect because it is a form of human life. Parness (1985) also wrote that the *Roe* decision "has been grossly misunderstood. Some have read it as a clear and sweeping rejection of the state's ability to protect previable, potential human life. The decision was not so sweeping" (p.103). Parness continued:

> Because the *Roe* decision suggested that the state's interest in protecting the
> potentiality of human life and in recognizing and respecting the humanity
> of the developing fetus was valid, the state may pursue those interests in the
> criminal law context. Specifically, the state may protect the potentiality of human
> life by punishing culpable conduct that harms the fetus and results in
> either death or disability. Additionally, the state may further its interest in
> according dignity to the unborn by creating sanctions for disrespectful conduct directed against the unborn (p.115).

Parness (1985) pointed out that many states require that fetal remains be disposed of in a considerate manner. Several states prohibit experimentation on fetuses except in cases in which the purpose of the research is to keep the fetus alive. These laws suggest that the fetus, under certain circumstances, receives the same treatment as humans that are born alive.

DEVELOPING RIGHTS

In the span of 100 years, the rights of the fetus have developed and expanded. Osborne (1984, p.707) wrote, "The child has gone from having no legal standing to being on the brink of having significant rights in its existence." But the courts have varied over the interpretation of the laws and their application. The rights of the fetus are emerging. A trend in case law has been to expand fetal rights; only in the area of criminal law have the embryo and the fetus not been treated the same as a child born alive (Goichman & Hirsh, 1984).

Although medical science is currently able to treat a small number of birth disorders *in utero,* for the overwhelming majority of disorders the only "treatment" is abortion.

Other chapters in this book will explore ethical views as well as the impact of new technologies on medical decisionmaking with respect to fetuses and infants at risk of developing severe disabilities.

REFERENCES

Albala v. City of New York, 429 N. E. 2d 1089 (N. Y., 1981).
Andrews, D.K. (1984). Recognizing a cause of action for preconception torts in light of medical and legal advancements regarding the unborn. *UMKC Law Review*, 53 (1), 78-07.
Beal, R. (1984). "Can I sue Mommy?" An analysis of a woman's tort liability for prenatal injuries to her child born alive. *San Diego Law Review*, 21, 325-370.
Bonbrest v. Kotz, 65 F.Supp 138 (1946).
California v. Smith, 129 Cal. Rptr. 498 (1976).
Cohen, L. G. (1986). Selective abortion and the diagnosis of fetal damage: Issues and concerns. *Journal of the Association for Persons with Severe Handicaps*, 11, 188-195.
Collins, (1983-84). An overview and analysis: prenatal torts, preconception torts, wrongful life, wrongful death, and wrongful birth: Time for a new framework. *Journal of Family Law*, 22, 677-709.
Commonwealth v. Cass, 467 N.E. 2d 1324 (Mass., 1984).
Curlender v. Bio-Science Laboratories, 106 Cal. App. 3d (1980).
Dietrich v. Inhabitants of Northampton, 52 Am. R. 242 (1884).
Doe v. Bolton, 410 U.S. 739 (1973).
Dunn v. Rose Way, Inc., 333 N.W. 2d 830 (1983).
Endresz v. Friedberg, 24 N.Y. 2d 478 (1969).
Feron, J. (1988, July 22). Surrender baby at birth, judge tells a woman. *The New York Times*, p.B2.
Gleitman v. Cosgrove, 227 A.2d 689 (1967).
Goichman, G., & Hirsh, H. L. (1984). The expanding rights of the fetus: An evolution not a revolution. *Medical Trial Technique Quarterly*, Fall, 212-230.
Jacob v. Theimer, 18 Tex. Sup. Ct. J. 222 (1975).
Jefferson v. Griffin Spalding County Hospital Authority, 274 S.E. 2d 457 (1981).
Jorgenson v. Meade Johnson Laboratories, 336 F.Supp. 961 (N.D. OKLA. 1972).
Kader, D. (1980). The law of tortious prenatal death since *Roe v. Wade*. *Missouri Law Review*, 45, 639-666.
Keeler v. Superior Court of Amador County, 470 Pacific Reporter 2d. 617 (Calif. 1970).
Kelly v. Gregory, 125 N.Y. Supp. 2d. 696 (1953).
Lewin, T. (1988, August 2). Protecting the baby: Work in pregnancy poses legal frontier. *The New York Times*, p.1, A15.
Life from Death. (1983, October 16). *The New York Times*, Sec. 1, p.41.
Louisiana v. Brown, 378 S. 2d 916 (La. 1979).
Manner, R. (1982). Court-ordered surgery for the protection of a viable fetus. *Western New England Law Review*, 5, 125-148.
McAuley v. Wills, 351 Ga. 3 (1983).
Osborne, K.R. (1984). Torts—The right of recovery for the tortious death of the unborn. *Howard Law Journal*, 27, 1649-1682.
Parness, J., (1985). Crimes against the unborn: Protecting and respecting the potentiality of human life. *Harvard Journal on Legislation*, 22, 97-172.
Parness, J. & Pritchard, S. (1982). To be or not to be: Protecting the unborn's potentiality of life. *University of Cincinnati Law Review*, 51 (2), 257-298.
Piper v. Hoard, 107 N.Y. 73 (1887).
Renslow v. Mennonite Hospital, 40 Ill. App 3d 234 (1977).
Rhoden, N. K. (1984). The new neonatal dilemma: Live births from late abortions. *Georgetown Law Journal*, 72, 1451-1509.
Roe v. Wade, 410 U.S. 113 (1973).
Ruling by a court keeps fetus alive. (1986, July 26). *The New York Times*, p.7.
Scofield, T. J. (1982). Recovery for the tortious death of the unborn. *South Carolina Law Review*, 33, 797-817.
Steinbock, B. (1986). The logical case for "wrongful life." *The Hastings Center Report*, 16, 15-20.
Stoutamire, S. S. (1981). The effect of legalized abortion on wrongful life actions. *Florida State University Law Review*, 9, 137-156.
Turpin v. Sortini, 182 Cal. Rptr. 337 (1982).
Verkennes v. Corniea, 38 N.W. 2d 838 (1949).
Webb, B. D. (1971). Is the intentional killing of an unborn child homocide? California's law to punish the willful killing of a fetus. *Pacific Law Journal*, 2(1), 170-185.
Zepeda v. Zepeda, 41 Ill App2d 240 (1963).

Chapter 2

Advances in Prenatal Diagnosis: Ethical Issues

For I was conceived after antibiotics yet before amniocentesis, late enough to have benefited from medicine's ability to prevent and control fetal infections, yet early enough to escape from medicine's ability to prevent me from living to suffer from my genetic disease (Singer, 1976, p.291).

Advances in research within the past few decades have led to significant developments in prenatal diagnosis. The diagnosis of a fetal disorder can help the family and the physician make an informed decision among alternatives: selective abortion; treatment of the fetus *in utero* through the use of transfusion, drug therapy, or surgery; special considerations regarding the delivery; transfer to specialized medical facility for the mother or for the newborn infant; treatment of the newborn; preparation for any special considerations that the birth of a child with a disability may require; or a decision not to intervene (Chervenak, Isaacson, & Mahoney, 1986).

Therapeutic abortion is the most controversial of these alternatives (U.S. Department of Health, Education, and Welfare, 1979). The number of abortions performed because of positive prenatal diagnostic test results is one-tenth of one percent of the total number of abortions performed in the U.S. (Tietze, 1984). Harrison, Golbus, and Filly (1981) listed fetal disorders and their management (see Table 2.1).

PRENATAL DIAGNOSTIC TECHNIQUES

Rapid developments in prenatal diagnosis occurred in the 1970s. Spurred on by the use of amniocentesis and legalized abortion, genetic counseling centers rapidly increased (Kevles, 1985). Kevles (1985), in his book *In the Name of Eugenics,* described the growth of genetic counseling centers. In 1960, there were only 30 to 40 centers in the United States. By 1970, there were about 400, with almost one quarter of them established and supported by the National Foundation–March of Dimes.

TABLE 2.1

Management of Fetal Malformations

Managed by Selective Abortion
Anencephaly, porencephaly, encephalocele, and giant hydrocephalus
Severe anomalies associated with chromosomal abnormalities (i.e., trisomy 13, trisomy 18)
Renal agenesis or bilateral polycystic kidney disease inherited chromosomal, metabolic, and
   hematologic abnormalities (e.g., hemoglobinopathies, Tay-Sachs disease)

Detectable *in Utero* but Best Corrected After Delivery at Term
Esophageal, duodenal, jejunoileal, and anorectal atresias
Meconium ileus (cystic fibrosis)
Enteric cysts and duplications
Small intact omphalocele
Small intact meningocele, myelomeningocele, and spina bifida
Unilateral multicystic dysplastic kidney
Craniofacial, extremity, and chest wall deformities
Cystic hygroma
Small sacrococcygeal teratoma
Ovarian cysts

May Require Induced Preterm Delivery for Early Correction *Ex Utero*
Obstructive hydronephrosis
Obstructive hydrocephalus
Amniotic band malformation complex
Gastroschsis or ruptured omphalocele
Intestinal ischemia-necrosis secondary to such conditions as volvvulus and meconium ileus
Hydrops fetalis
Intrauterine growth retardation

May Require Cesarean Delivery
Conjoined twins
Giant omphalocele, ruptured omphalocele/gastroschisis
Large hydrocephalus
Large sacrcoccygeal teratoma
Large cystic hygroma
Large or ruptured meningomyelocele
Malformations requiring preterm delivery in the presence of inadequate labor or fetal distress

May Require Treatment *in Utero*
Deficiency states that may be alleviated
Deficient pulmonary surfactant (pulmonary immaturity)
Anemia-erythroblastosis and hydrops
Hypothyroidism and goiter
Methylmalonic acidemia
(B12-dependent)
Multiple carboxylase deficiency (biotin-dependent)
Nutritional deficiency and intrauterine growth retardation
Anatomic lesions that interfere with development
Bilateral hydronephrosis (urethral obstruction)
Diaphragmatic hernia
Obstructive hydrocephalus

From: Harrison, Golbus, & Filly (1981). Reprinted by permission.

Strong pressure for research in genetics has come from persons with genetic disorders and their families. Numerous organizations, including the National Genetics Foundation, the Hereditary Disease Foundation, the National Hemophilia Foundation, the Cooley's Anemia Foundation, the Cystic Fibrosis Foundation, and the Huntington's Disease Foundation of America, support research and lobby on behalf of affected persons. These organizations "welcome the powerful new tools for prenatal diagnosis emerging from the accelerating advance of biomedical knowledge and techniques" (Kelves, 1985, p.293).

Prenatal diagnostic techniques, which are used to determine the presence of chromosomal, metabolic, or structural defects in the fetus, are frequently employed medical procedures. There are two outcomes of positive identification of fetal defects: a) the continuity of the normal and desired pregnancy in which the well-being of the mother and fetus are the major concerns (Campbell, 1979); and b) the treatment and cure of disorders in the fetus and the infant (Powledge & Fletcher, 1979). Amniocentesis, fetoscopy, ultrasound imaging techniques, alphafetoprotein screening, and chorionic villus sampling provide information to the parents and the physician about the fetus and may be used to decide whether, if the technology is available, to treat the fetus *in utero* or after birth or whether to terminate the pregnancy.

Prenatal diagnosis raises a number of ethical, legal, social, and psychological issues that have been "thrown in high relief by recent developments" (Neel, 1971, p.219).

Amniocentesis

Amniocentesis is a medical diagnostic procedure that is widely used to determine the presence of chromosomal or metabolic disorders in the fetus. Since at least 1881, when the first known use of needles was introduced into the uterus, amniocentesis has been a method of diagnosis of fetal disorders (Milunsky, 1979a).

However, it was not until the 1950s that amniocentesis became a routine diagnostic test. Since the first reports of its use, the number of amniocentesis procedures has increased rapidly (Smith, 1981).

Numerous conditions can be diagnosed using this procedure (Babson, Pernoll, & Benda, 1980; Harrison, Golbus, & Filly, 1981), including Down syndrome, anencephaly, encephalocele, hydrocephalus, Tay-Sachs disease, glycogen storage diseases, maple syrup urine disease, Niemann-Pick disease, galactosemia, and Lesch-Nyan syndrome.

This list and the ones that follow are partial ones because the number of disorders that can be diagnosed through prenatal diagnostic techniques is large and progress in genetic research is leading to a rapid increase in the number of identifiable conditions.

Amniocentesis is usually performed between the 14th and 16th weeks of pregnancy on an outpatient basis. After the injection of a local anesthetic, a needle is inserted into the skin, through the uterine wall and into the amniotic fluid. The fluid sample is then withdrawn.

Frequently, this procedure is accompanied by the use of ultrasound techniques that assist the physician in placing the needle correctly and determining gestational age (U.S. Department of Health, Education, and Welfare, 1979). Results take several weeks and may cause the decision to have an abortion to be delayed, thus raising the possibility of additional problems.

If chromosomal or metabolic disorders are found to be present in the fetus, the parents and physician use this information to decide whether to abort or treat the fetus (if treatment is a possibility) or whether to not intervene at all.

Smith (1981) and Hansen (1978) found that for Down syndrome, a condition that can be detected through the use of amniocentesis and for which there is no medical treatment, the number of abortions has increased. Approximately 10% of second trimester abortions are performed on women who find out as a result of the amniocentesis that they are carrying a fetus with a disorder (Kleiman, 1984).

Fetoscopy

Although amniocentesis provides "a window to the fetus" (Mahoney & Hobbins, 1979, p.501), amniotic fluid and amniotic cells contain limited information about the genetic and metabolic condition of the fetus. Fetoscopy, which was developed in the 1950s, (U.S. Department of Health, Education, and Welfare, 1979) is a technique that permits visualization of the fetus *in utero* through an endoscope and also allows the sampling of fetal tissue and blood. Mahoney and Hobbins (1979) recommended that fetoscopy be conducted between the 15th and 20th weeks of pregnancy.

The fetoscopy procedure involves the application of a local anesthetic on the abdomen of the pregnant woman, making a small incision, and inserting an endoscope. A sample of fetal tissue and blood can then be taken (U.S. Department of Health, Education, and Welfare, 1979).

Many diagnoses, especially anatomical abnormalities, can be made almost immediately. Direct viewing of the fetus allows diagnosis of Ellis-van Crevald syndrome, trisomy 13, and spina bifida. Among the diseases that can be identified through the use of the fetal blood sample are beta-thalassemia, sickle cell anemia, chronic granulomatous disease, and classic hemophilia (U.S. Department of Health, Education, and Welfare, 1979).

Ultrasonography

Ultrasound imaging techniques transmit high-frequency, low-intensity sound waves through the woman's abdomen. As the sound waves pass through maternal and fetal tissues, they are reflected back and are eventually transformed into visual images on a screen. The fetal images are in two dimensions and not all of the fetus, such as the limbs, fingers and toes, can always be viewed.

Although many researchers have found that ultrasonography is not hazardous, there is some research that indicates that it may produce pathological results (U. S. Department of Health, Education and Welfare, 1979). Virtually all pregnant women undergo this technique as part of routine prenatal care (Campbell, 1979).

There are several different types of ultrasound (Blatt, 1988). Level One ultrasound generates one or two-dimensional pictures that can be used to estimate the fetal age, weight, placental location, and fetal body parts. Level Two ultrasound shows the movements of the fetus such as heartbeat, breathing, arm and leg movements, and swallowing. The third type, Doppler ultrasound, measures fetal heart rate and heart sound. Some of the conditions that can be detected using ultrasound techniques include anencephaly, encephalocele, meningomyelocele, hydrocephaly, porencehaly, renal dysplasia, duodenal atresia, and duodneal atresia (U. S. Department of Health, Education and Welfare, 1979).

The accuracy of ultrasonography seems to depend on the potential diagnosis that will be made. In a study of the use of ultrasound techniques and the diagnosis of anencephaly in 100 cases, Chervenak, Farley, Walters, Hobbins, and Mahoney (1984) found that no false positive diagnoses were made. But microcephaly, cleft lip, and other diagnoses are more difficult to make just on the basis of ultrasound techniques (Chervenak, Isaacson, & Mahoney, 1986).

In addition to diagnosing fetal damage, ultrasound imaging can be used with amniocentesis to locate the placenta and the fetus, identify multiple pregnancies, determine the age of the fetus, study the development of a fetus with a disorder, diagnose growth or structural abnormalities in the fetus, identify changes in the volume of amniotic fluid, assist in fetal surgery *in utero*, and confirm fetal death (Blatt, 1988; Campbell, 1979; Chervenak, Isaacson, & Mahoney, 1986).

Alphafetoprotein Screening

In the 1970s, several researchers discovered that elevated levels of fetal serum alphafetoprotein (AFP) can be measured in the mother's blood between 16 and 18 weeks of pregnancy (U.S. Department of Health, Education, and Welfare, 1979). AFP is a fetal globulin that occurs in the fetal urine and is deposited into the amniotic fluid (Milunsky, 1979b).

Elevated levels of serum alphafetoprotein have been associated with twins, Down syndrome, neural tube defects (NTD), anencephaly, hydrocephaly, fetal death, and ventral wall defects.

AFP testing is only an initial step in prenatal screening and if the results are positive, ultrasonography will be conducted. Based on the results of this test, amniocentesis may be recommended. In the United States, amniocentesis is usually accompanied by AFP screening (President's Commission for the Study of Ethical Problems, 1983).

There are many causes of NTDs, some of which are known, and others for which there is no known cause. Because the only groups thus far identified at high risk for NTD are women with a family history of NTD, it has been recommended that all women undergo AFP screening.

Chorionic Villus Sampling

Although amniocentesis is used to satisfactorily detect chromosomal and genetic disorders in the fetus, its major disadvantages are that it cannot be performed until at least the 14th week of pregnancy and it may take several weeks for results to be obtained. For women who receive positive results and decide to terminate the pregnancy, the decision to have an abortion is not made until well into the second trimester. Chorionic villus sampling can be performed much earlier in the pregnancy.

Chorionic villus sampling can be used to aid in the diagnosis of chromosome-related defects, such as Down syndrome, cystic fibrosis, and sick-cell anemia, and metabolic and biochemical disorders, such as Tay-Sachs disease. In addition, it can be used to determine the gender of the fetus, but it cannot be used in the diagnosis of neural tube defects (Blatt, 1988).

Chorionic villus sampling is a surgical technique that removes tissue from the uterus. A piece of chorion, the outer tissue of the sac that surrounds the fetus is removed using a catheter that is inserted through the vagina (Blatt, 1988; Jackson, 1985).

In a relatively new technique that is similar to amniocentesis, a needle is inserted into the abdomen and a sample of the chorion is removed. Results can be obtained within a few hours and, if abortion is a consideration, it can be performed during the first trimester when it is safer and easier to do so. The risks of this technique are similar to those associated with amniocentesis (Jackson, 1985). Complications include infection, septic shock bleeding, fetal injury, cervical tears,and miscarriage (Blatt, 1988; Rhoads et al., 1989).

While chorionic villus sampling has several important advantages over amniocentesis, there are some significant drawbacks. Because the research on this procedure is relatively recent, much more information is needed to evaluate the risks of miscarriage. Laboratory procedures for the analysis are still being refined and established. Neural tube defects cannot be diagnosed with this procedure and fetal anatomy cannot be viewed (Blakemore, 1988). In addition, there seems to be higher chance of inconclusive diagnoses and procedure failures (Rhoads et al., 1989).

Other Prenatal Diagnostic Tests

Cell sorting, fetal skin sampling, gene probe tests, and percutaneous umbilical blood sampling are four prenatal diagnostic procedures that are still experimental. Because it is known that a few fetal cells enter the mother's circulatory system, a new laser technology procedure has been developed that involves sorting the fetal cells from the mother's cells.

Another test, which uses fetoscopy, involves the sampling of fetal skin in order to detect rare skin disorders. Gene probe tests are used with samples of chorionic villi that have been obtained through chorionic villus sampling. Through the use of DNA testing, hereditary conditions such as cystic fibrosis, Huntington's disease, hemophilia, and Duchenne muscular dystrophy can be diagnosed (Blatt, 1988).

Percutaneous umbilical blood sampling (PUBS) is an experimental technique that samples fetal blood. A needle is inserted through the abdomen and into the umbilical vein (the umbilical cord contains two arteries and one vein). PUBS can be used to diagnose many of the same conditions as amniocentesis (Blatt, 1988). Although this is still an experimental procedure, it has been reported that PUBS is very accurate (Blatt, 1988).

ETHICAL ISSUES

The widespread use of prenatal diagnostic techniques, their accuracy and effectiveness, as well as the rapid advances in research raise significant ethical issues. The urgent task "of establishing an ethics of use for their widely accumulating knowledge and biotechnical power" (Kevles, 1985, p.301) awaits us. Many of the advances go beyond current legal and ethical standards, with developments in technology far outstripping current ethical standards. In this section, some of the ethical issues are presented.

Two of the most fundamental and highly publicized and politicized issues relating to prenatal diagnosis are the point at which life begins and the moral status of the fetus. Because these issues have been widely discussed on television and the radio, in the popular press, and in scholarly publications they will not be repeated here. Rather, the focus will concern the ethical issues that surround the diagnosis of a fetal disorder. Numerous authors have written about the ethical issues surrounding prenatal diagnosis. Representative writers and their viewpoints will be presented.

Normality and Abnormality—The Degrading of Society

Ramsey (1973) believed that prenatal diagnosis should be limited in its use. He approved of prenatal screening only for contagious diseases that the fetus may have and only if treatment can be provided if the fetus is found to have a disorder. Otherwise, "amniocentesis is ethically most problematic if, indeed, it is not to be morally censured" (Ramsey, 1973, p.148).

Ramsey opposed prenatal screening because the results of the screening can "degrade society's willingness to accept and care for abnormal children and, at the same time, to enlarge the category of unacceptable abnormality, while narrowing the range of acceptable normality" (Ramsey, 1973, p.148). He argued that fetuses that do not meet certain standards of normality will be classified as abnormal and that individuals must meet certain societal standards in order to have a life "worth living and to be deserving of care in the human community" (Ramsey, 1973, p.148).

One consequence of amniocentesis is to narrow the concept of normality and therefore entail the "degrading of care for human abnormality" (Ramsey, 1973, p.160). Society, if held to these standards, will be demeaned. In order to avoid these problems, Ramsey opposed prenatal diagnosis and proposed:

> that an individual shall not be certified to be among us—counted equally—until two days after birth, or when he can have his first 'check-up' to determine whether he can qualify for the 'quality of life' we mean to enhance (1973, p.160).

Kass (1973) also supported Ramsey's position. Kass based his views on "the belief in the radical moral equality of all human beings, the belief that all human beings possess equally and independent of merit certain fundamental rights, one among which is, of course, the right to life" (Kass, 1973, p.187). But Kass was also very concerned about society's attitudes toward persons who may be disabled. While both Ramsey's and Kass' views seem to be patronizing toward persons with disabilities, they are important. Kass believed that negative attitudes toward persons with disabilities devalues all of us:

> How will we come to view and act toward the many 'abnormals' that will remain among us—the retarded, the crippled, the senile, the deformed, and the true mutants (sic)—once we embark on a program to root out genetic abnormals—some who escape detection or whose disease is undetectable *in utero,* others as a result of new mutations, birth injuries, accidents, maltreatment, or disease—who will require our care and protection. The existence of 'defectives' cannot be fully prevented, not even by totalitarian breeding and weeding programs. Is it not likely that our principle with respect to these people will change from 'We try harder' to 'Why accept second best?' The idea of 'the unwanted because abnormal child' may become a self-fulfilling prophecy, whose consequences may be worse than those of the abnormality itself (1973, p.190).

Opposing these views, Morison (1973) wrote that society will be "in danger if we don't accept abortion as one means of ensuring that both the quantity and quality of the human race are kept within reasonable limits" (Morison, 1973, pp.210-211). He compared society's interest in the number of children that are born with the quality of these children. His idea of what it means for a child to have "quality" is not well defined.

Writing that society has a legitimate interest in the "quality" of children, Morison stated:

> Now, when a defective child may cost the society many thousands of dollars a year for a whole lifetime without returning the benefit, it would appear inevitable that society should do what it reasonably can to assure that those children who are born can lead normal and reasonably independent lives. It goes without saying that if the model couple is to be restricted to 2.1 children, it is also more important to them that all their children be normal than it was when an abnormal child was, in effect, diluted by a large number of normal siblings. And the over-all point here again is that the interests of society and the interests of the family become coincident at this stage, when they both realize that there are a limited number of slots to be filled (1973, p.208).

Eugenic Uses of Prenatal Diagnosis

Fletcher (1979, 1983), while supporting selective abortion "in medically severe cases for which there is no therapy" (1979, p.626), was concerned about the eugenic uses of prenatal diagnosis. With advances in medical technology, the accuracy and efficiency of prenatal diagnostic techniques will continue to improve; Fletcher wondered whether "campaigns might be mounted to 'attack' disorders like Down syndrome, Huntington's disease, or cystic fibrosis" (Fletcher, 1983, p.147). Pressure could be placed on targeted groups to comply with recommended prenatal diagnostic screening procedures because the costs of selectively aborting a fetus with a disorder is cheaper than caring for a child who is disabled:

> A climate of moral blame may be cast around parents who did not comply. In such a climate, those who live and cope with the burdens of genetic disorders may feel more demeaned and compelled to counter the pressure on them and their descendants 'to be eugenically responsible' with moral claims of their own fair treatment and restraint from punishment (1983, p.148).

Thompson (1979) pointed out that the effects of prenatal diagnosis can be eugenically neutral, dysgenic, or eugenic. As an example, Thompson explained that abortion of a fetus with Tay-Sachs disease would have a neutral effect on the gene pool because children who are born with Tay-Sachs disease do not live long enough to reproduce. But parents who carry the gene for Tay-Sachs disease may choose only to have children who have been identified through the use of prenatal diagnosis and are not affected. These unaffected children may be carriers of the Tay-Sachs gene and, thus, additional carriers of the gene may be the dysgenic result. A eugenic benefit would be the selective abortion of affected fetuses because the costs of the medical care of these children would be saved.

According to Thompson, in policy decisions involving prenatal diagnosis there is little value in determining the effects on the gene pool because the effects over succeeding generations is very small. "These effects are, however, so exiguous—the small probability that a given carrier will mate with another (or an affected homozygote with a carrier) weighted more negligibly by discounting to present value over the span of a generation—as not to merit consideration" (Thompson, 1979, p.642).

Even for Huntington's chorea, the gene pool effects are minimal. Thompson, while seeming to support the abortion of fetuses with severe disorders, was concerned about the abortion of fetuses with mild genetic disorders. He did, to a certain extent agree with Fletcher, when he wrote that individuals who have genetic disorders or parents who carry the gene for these orders may become stigmatized. "If we abort or avoid the births of individuals with minimally disabling genetic diseases (actions not justified by concern for the burdens placed on parents or on public institutions), we risk stigmatizing those carrying or affected with such conditions" (Thompson, 1979, p.642).

Social Policies

Milunsky and Fletcher (1978) addressed the ethical issues relating to the formation of social policies for genetic screening using prenatal diagnostic techniques. As the ability to diagnose genetic diseases increases, programs that identify genetic carriers of certain diseases, that provide care for pregnant women, and that offer selective abortion will have to be designed. One ethical issue that arises is whether to extend the services that are already available in private clinics (e.g., information and education, genetic screening, abortion) to a broader group of women. If only women who are able to afford the services of a private clinic are the ones who use the services, then the issue of equal access is important.

A second ethical issue identified by Milunsky and Fletcher (1978) was who determines what kind of human beings should be born. What kinds of influence should counselors and physicians have in determining genetic health? They believed that two different attitudes could emerge here.

The first is that reproduction should be controlled in order to prevent the birth of persons with disorders. The second attitude is that "one should avoid suffering wherever possible, but with the knowledge that there are vital interest groups involved in the definition of disease and human health" (Milunsky & Fletcher, 1978, p.1344).

The third ethical issue is how the screening program will treat abortion:

> Will the program be designed, for example, with the assumption that one ought to abort in each case for Down's syndrome or that abortion will be presented as an option with no recognition of the moral problems? How will a couple be treated who desire to accept an infant with Down's syndrome

following positive diagnosis and confirmation of the disorder? (Milunsky & Fletcher, 1978, p.1344).

For each of these ethical dilemmas, Milunsky and Fletcher (1978) seemed to argue for tolerance, debate, and inclusion of diverse viewpoints:

> A voluntary and pluralistic social policy of genetic screening and prenatal diagnosis will protect the greatest range of values—access to health care, promotion of genetic health, freedom of decision, and the right to reproduce—for those who continue to find abortion the greatest problem associated with prenatal diagnosis (p.1345).

In 1989, in a major policy shift, the U.S. Public Health Service recommended that less prenatal care be extended to pregnant women whose fetuses were not at risk. A panel of experts determined that women whose babies were at risk of prematurity or low birthweight should be given additional attention. The panel felt that many routine tests, such as screening for protein in the urine, routine blood pressure tests, and more than one pelvic examination were expensive, time consuming, and of questionable benefit to healthy pregnant women. Although the panel did not determine the cost savings relating to the care of healthy pregnant women, it recommended that pregnant women who were at risk provided with help including information about proper nutrition, the risks of smoking, the risks of drugs and alcohol, as well as assistance with problems that might lead to child abuse (Kolata, 1989).

Unanswered Questions

Many unanswered questions remain. How many defects make a fetus a candidate for an abortion? Should a fetus with a cleft palate, which can be corrected with one operation, be aborted? The Genetics Research Group of The Hastings Center recommended that physicians resuscitate and treat babies born after an attempted abortion (Powledge & Fletcher 1979). Should the same technology that is used to treat premature newborns also be used to treat aborted fetuses that, although injured during the abortion process, survive late abortions? If fetal disorders are correctable, should physicians be required to perform abortions?

Harrison, Golbus, and Filly (1981) raised other questions:

> Who makes decisions for the fetus? How can the risk of intervention be weighed against the burden of malformation itself? For example, a mother carrying a fetus with urethral obstruction and severe bilateral hydronephrosis must weigh the risk of correction against not only the risk of neonatal death or severe disability from renal or pulmonary failure, but also the emotional and financial burden of prolonged arduous, expensive, and sometimes unrewarding treatment of chronic renal failure. The lifelong emotional and

financial burden of any given malformation on the person and his family should be weighed against the risk of fetal intervention undertaken to ameliorate this burden (1981, p.777).

Milunsky and Fletcher (1978) raised still more questions:

When the prenatal test cannot distinguish affected from unaffected males—as at the present time—should all males be aborted? Should the parents live with the consequences? In the case of muscular dystrophy, what do parents do with the fact that affected males will be normal for the first few years of life? Since females carry the gene that communicates these diseases, should the female fetus be allowed to live and magnify the problem in the future? (p.1343).

GUIDELINES FOR PRENATAL
DIAGNOSIS

Powledge and Fletcher (1979), in a report of the Genetics Research Group of The Hastings Center, addressed many of the concerns about prenatal diagnosis in a set of guidelines "for the development and institutionalization of prenatal diagnostic programs and to help workers in this area provide the most favorable circumstances for thoughtful, informed, morally responsible decision making by parents" (p.169). The report discussed the following eighteen guidelines:

1. Prenatal diagnostic programs should be devised to target groups of pregnant women who are at risk.
2. Prenatal diagnosis should be made available only when excellent laboratory services can be provided. Even though error rates are low, there are ethical and legal consequences relating to inaccurate results. Likewise, high quality control standards must be maintained as well as training for laboratory employees.
3. The lowest possible error rates must be set. In many cases, a positive test will result in an abortion and a negative test may result in the birth of a child with a handicap or potential handicap. When a positive test is made, additional tests may be necessary to confirm it.
4. Both short-term and long-term follow-up activities must be initiated in order to determine the effects of a prenatal diagnosis.
5. Adequate information should be provided to the parents before the prenatal diagnostic procedure is undertaken. The risks involved, side effects, and any consequences of the procedure must be explained.
6. The privacy of the patient (the mother, and, in many cases, the father) must be preserved. Although genetic registries and data banks are important, scrupulous care must be given to maintaining privacy and confidentiality.
7. The provision of prenatal diagnostic techniques in a physician's office

should not lead to a lowering of the standards of quality control or to a lessening of the need for confidentiality, privacy, and counseling.

8. There should be a clear difference between the provision of prenatal diagnosis for research purposes and the provision of prenatal diagnosis for routine services to selected groups of pregnant women. When used experimentally, the patients must be made aware of the experimental nature and the risks of the procedures.

9. Women who have decided not to have an abortion should not be denied access to prenatal diagnosis. The knowledge that a fetus is free from any disorders can be a great relief.

10. Counseling for prenatal diagnosis should respect parental feelings about abortion. The counseling should not be coercive.

11. Parents should be informed about all possibilities for disorders in which prenatal diagnosis and treatment are available. Although treatment may be available, some families may decide not to continue with the pregnancy because they do not want to have a child who has that disorder.

12. Prenatal determination of the sex of the fetus should be available when other techniques for the diagnosis of sex-linked disorders are not available. High priority should be given to research on the prenatal identification of these disorders.

13. Information about various disorders should not be withheld from the parents even when the knowledge about these disorders seems to be of questionable value.

14. The use of prenatal diagnostic techniques solely for the determination of the sex of the fetus should be discouraged.

15. If a live birth occurs after an attempt is made to abort the fetus, standard procedures relating to resuscitation and treatment of newborns should be practiced. These newborns should be considered critically ill and decisionmaking should follow the guidelines and procedures that have been developed for these infants.

16. Treatment decisions for critically ill newborns should not be based on the prenatal diagnosis. The prenatal diagnosis should not provide the rationale for withholding treatment and services from infants.

17. Third-party payments such as Medicaid should be permitted. Pregnant women of lower socioeconomic levels should have access to prenatal diagnostic techniques.

18. The benefits of prenatal diagnosis should be publicized by "the government, the medical profession, major foundations, and voluntary health agencies. This communication effort should be aimed at both professionals and consumers, but at a pace that does not create greater demand than existing services can safely meet" (Powledge & Fletcher, 1979, p.172).

ON A COLLISION COURSE WITH
THE FUTURE

As suggested in the beginning, this chapter has been directed toward a discussion of the issues rather than their solution. Are we, by default, permitting advances in technology to determine our future policies? Fletcher (1983) wrote:

Unless present trends change, in the next few years the public will see earlier and safer methods of prenatal diagnosis combined with more efficacious methods of fetal therapy. For some time to come, the power to diagnose will far outstrip the power to treat, but with sufficient research and resources, the two activities of fetal medicine will assume more balance (p.156).

REFERENCES

Babson, S. G., Pernoll, M. L., & Benda, G. I. (1980). *Diagnosis and management of the fetus and neonate at risk*. St. Louis: C. V. Mosby.
Blakemore, K. J. (1988). Prenatal diagnosis by chorionic villus sampling. *Obstetrics and Gynecology Clinics of North America, 15,* 179-213.
Blatt, R. J. R. (1988). *Prenatal Tests.* New York: Vintage Books.
Campbell, S. (1979). Diagnosis of fetal abnormalities by ultrasound. In A. Milunsky (Ed.), *Genetic disorders and the fetus* (pp.431-467). New York: Plenum.
Chervenak, F. A., Farley, M. A., Walters, L., Hobbins, J. C., & Mahoney, M. J. (1984). When is termination of pregnancy during the third trimester morally justifiable? *The New England Journal of Medicine, 310,* 501-504.
Chervenak, F.A., Isaacson, G., & Mahoney, M.J. (1986). Advances in the diagnosis of fetal defects. *The New England Journal of Medicine, 315,* 305-307.
Fletcher, J. C. (1979). The morality and ethics of prenatal diagnosis. In A. Milunsky (Ed.), *Genetic disorders and the fetus* (pp.621-635). New York: Plenum.
Fletcher, J. C. (1983). Ethics and trends in applied human genetics. *Birth Defects, 19,* 143-158.
Hansen, H. (1978). Decline of Down's syndrome after abortion reform in New York state. *American Journal of Mental Deficiency, 83,* 185-188.
Harrison, M., Golbus, M., & Filly, R. (1981). Management of the fetus with a correctable congenital defect. *Journal of the American Medical Association, 246,* 774-777.
Jackson, L.G. (1985). First-trimester diagnosis of fetal disorders. *Hospital Practice, 20,* 39-48.
Kass, L. R. (1973). Implications of prenatal diagnosis for the human right to life. In B. Hilton, D. Callahan, M. Harris, P. Condliffe, & B. Berkley (Eds.), *Ethical issues in human genetics* (pp.185-199). New York: Plenum.
Kevles, D. J. (1985). *In the name of eugenics.* New York: Alfred A. Knopf.
Kleiman, D. (1984, February 15). When abortion becomes birth: A dilemma of medical ethics shaken by new advances. *The New York Times,* p.B1.
Kolata, G. (1989, October 4). Less prenatal care urged for most healthy women. *The New York Times,* pp.A1, A22.
Mahoney, M. J., & Hobbins, J. C. (1979). Fetoscopy and fetal blood sampling. In A. Milunsky (Ed.), *Genetic disorders and the fetus* (pp.501-526). New York: Plenum.
Milunsky, A. (1979a). Amniocentesis. In A. Milunsky (Ed.), *Genetic disorders and the fetus* (pp.19-46). New York: Plenum.
Milunsky, A. (1979b). Prenatal diagnosis of neural tube defects. In A. Milunsky (Ed.), *Genetic disorders and the fetus* (pp.379-430). New York: Plenum
Milunsky, A., & Fletcher, J. C. (1978). Prenatal diagnosis. In W. T. Reich (Ed.), *Encyclopedia of Bioethics,* Vol. 3 (pp.1332-1346). New York: Free Press.

Morison, R. S. (1973). Implications of prenatal diagnosis for the quality of, and right to human life: Society as a standard. In B. Hilton, D. Callahan, M. Harris, P. Condliffe, & B. Berkley (Eds.), *Ethical issues in human genetics* (pp.201-211). New York: Plenum.

Neel, J. V. (1971). Ethical issues resulting from prenatal diagnosis. In M. Harris (Ed.), *Early diagnosis of human genetic defects: Scientific and ethical considerations* (pp.219-229). Bethesda, MD: NIH Publication (NIH 72-25).

Powledge, T. M., & Fletcher, J. (1979). Guidelines for the ethical, social and legal issues in prenatal diagnosis. *The New England Journal of Medicine, 300,* 168-172.

President's Commission for the Study of Ethical Problems in Medicine and Biomedical and Behavioral Research (1983). *Screening and counseling for genetic conditions.* Washington, D C: U.S. Government Printing Office.

Ramsey, P. (1973). Screening: an ethicist's view. In B. Hilton, D. Callahan, M. Harris, P. Condliffe, & B. Berkley (Eds.), *Ethical issues in human genetics* (pp.147-161). New York: Plenum.

Rhoads, G. G., Jackson, L. G., Schlesselman, E. E., de la Cruz, F. F., Desnick, R. J., Golbus, M. S., Ledbetter, D. H., Lubs, H. A., Mahoney, M. J., Pergament, E., Simpson, J. L., Carpenter, R. J., Elias, S., Ginsberg, N. A., Goldberg, J. D., Hobbins, J. C., Lunch, L., Shiono, P. H., Wapner, R. J., & Zachary, J. (1989). The safety and efficacy of chorionic villus sampling for early prenatal diagnosis of cytogenetic abnormalities. *The New England Journal of Medicine, 320,* 609-617.

Singer, J. D. (1976). Ethical and social problems of prenatal diagnosis. *Inserm, 61,* 291-297.

Smith, D. J. (1981). Down's Syndrome, amniocentesis and abortion: Prevention or elimination? *Mental Retardation, 19,* 8-11.

Thompson, M. S. (1979). Prenatal diagnosis and public policy. In A. Milunsky (Ed.), *Genetic disorders and the fetus* (pp.637-660). New York: Plenum.

Tietze, C. (1984). The public health effects of legal abortion in the United States. *Family Planning Perspectives, 16,* 26-28.

U.S. Department of Health, Education, and Welfare (1979). *Antenatal diagnosis.* (NIH Publication No. 79-1973). Bethesda, MD: National Institutes of Health.

Chapter 3

Selective Abortion: Social, Legal and Ethical Perspectives

Since 1967, the first year in which a state liberalized its abortion laws, more than 15 million abortions have been performed in the United States. A majority of the legal abortions that have been carried out have most likely replaced the abortions that had once been performed illegally. The rest have replaced unwanted or mistimed pregnancies. With the legalization of abortion, the number of women who have died because of abortions has significantly decreased, as did the number of women who would have suffered complications because of an abortion (Tietze, 1984).

Abundant information is available on the who, when, and why of abortion—who gets abortions, why women undergo abortions, and when abortions are performed. Approximately 1.6 million abortions are performed each year (McLouglin, 1988). The Alan Guttmacher Institute of New York projected that for every 100 women in the U. S., there will be 76 abortions (Kolata, 1988a). Since the 1973 *Roe v. Wade* decision, abortion rates in the United States have increased.

Regionally, the eastern and western states have the highest rates, the midwestern and southern states the lowest (Henry & Harvey, 1982). Eighty percent of these abortions are performed on unmarried women; twice as many nonwhite women received abortions as white women. Most of the women are under the age of 25; two out of every five women who have abortions have had previous abortions (McLouglin, 1988).

In two surveys conducted by the Alan Guttmacher Institute (Kolata, 1988b), women reported that they had abortions for a variety of reasons and most women gave more than one reason for having an abortion. Many women said that they had abortions because they did not have enough money or because they felt that a baby would interfere with their education or their work.

With respect to infants with disabilities, the legalization of abortion has had the effect of preventing the birth of an unknown number of infants who would have been disabled. The number of abortions performed because of positive prenatal diagnostic test results in 1982 was 1,500, or one tenth of one

Parts of this chapter were adapted from: Cohen, L. (1986). Selective abortion and the diagnosis of fetal damage: Issues and concerns. *The Journal of the Association for Persons with Severe Handicaps, 11,* 188-195.

percent of the total number of abortions performed in the U.S. during that year (Tietze, 1984). One poll of women's attitudes toward abortion ("Abortion," 1981) found that 87% of the women who were surveyed approved of abortion if the fetus had a genetic disorder. (Further, 92% approved if the woman's health were at risk; 88% approved if the woman had been raped; 79% if the woman were physically handicapped; and 72% if the mother were an unmarried teenager).

The *Encyclopedia of Bioethics* (Reich, 1978) included a definition of abortion as:

> Termination of pregnancy, spontaneously or by induction, prior to viability. Thereafter termination of pregnancy is called delivery. To the lay public the term spontaneous abortion is usually referred to as miscarriage. Induced abortions have been classified as therapeutic and nontherapeutic in the past, the terms often being used synonymously with legal and illegal abortion respectively. An induced termination of pregnancy prior to viability is not always regarded as an abortion in common parlance. For example, salpingectomy (removal of a fallopian tube) for ectopic pregnancy (pregnancy implanted in the tube) is a common, indeed, a universal practice...Similarly, most diagnostic uterine curettages are performed in the late stages of the menstrual cycle, when a fertilized ovum may well be present in the tube...(Hellegers, 1978, pp.2-3).

CONTEXTUAL ISSUES

The issue of selective or therapeutic abortion of a fetus with a disability or a potential disability is difficult to separate from the issue of abortion. The issue of abortion has given way to intense debate and Americans are deeply divided. One poll (Dionne, 1989) found that 49% of Americans favored keeping abortion legal, but that 39% believed that abortions should only be performed when there was rape, incest, or the mother's life was in danger; 9% wanted all abortions to be illegal.

In the United States, the issue of abortion has become politicized. Luker (1984a, b) interviewed 212 individuals who were identified as activists in the abortion arena. Using this limited sample, she concluded that the "world views" of these activists differed from one another. Persons who generally are not opposed to abortion are thought to be "pro-choice"; and persons who generally oppose abortion are thought to be "pro-life." These two groups, although not mutually exclusive or homogeneous, differ in how they view the world in general, and abortion is just one area in which they differ.

According to Luker (1984a, b), pro-life persons believe that because women and men are different from one another they have different roles in society. Pro-life persons hold the view that the embryo is a person. Embryos are human, at least at the genetic level, and therefore are entitled to all the rights to which humans are entitled. Pro-life persons are offended by the Supreme

Court's ruling in *Roe v. Wade* that a fetus is not a person. For them, the fetus *is* a person and no personal decision can affect this belief.

For pro-choice persons, moral considerations against killing do not apply to fetuses (Warren, 1978). The decision whether or not to have a child is weighed against competing arguments, which may include the availability of financial resources, the career demands of the woman, the number of children in the family, and religious beliefs. Thus, the decision whether or not to have an abortion is a necessary option best left to the individual. For these persons, a good parent is one who can provide more than love and care for children. A good parent considers the "emotional, psychological, social, and financial resources" (Luker, 1984a, p.181) necessary to raise a child.

Pro-life and pro-choice persons are very unlike each other. They differ considerably with respect to financial resources, educational levels, and occupations. These differences contribute to the choices of a mate and to their beliefs and values about family life (Luker, 1984a). Representative comments of the interviewees are included here.

Pro-life persons as cited by Luker (1984a) stated:

(Men and women) were created differently and we're meant to complement each other, and when you get away from our (proper) roles as such, you start obscuring them...(p.160).

I believe that there's a natural mother's instinct. And I'm kind of chauvinist this way, but I don't believe men and women are equal. I believe men and women are very different, and beautifully different, and that they're complementary in their nature to one another...(p.160).

One of the problems (of abortion), I think, is the further degradation of women in society. I know that feminists would disagree with me on this, and I consider myself a feminist, so it's difficult for me to relate to other feminists on this issue. I think having an abortion as an alternative—as a way out, I guess—makes it easier for men to exploit women than ever before...(p.162).

I think it's quite clear that the IUD is abortifacient 100 percent of the time and the pill is sometimes an abortifacient—it's hard to know just when, so I think we need to treat it as an abortifacient. It's not really that much of an issue with me, (but) I think there's a respect for germinal life that is equivalent to a respect for individual life...(p.165).

Representative views of pro-choice persons cited in Luker (1984a) include:

I just feel that one of the main reasons women have been in a secondary position culturally is because of the natural way things happen. Women would bear children because they had no way to prevent it, except by having no sexual involvement...(p.176).

I would say that the tip of the iceberg is purposeful parenthood. I think life is too cheap, I think we're too easy-going. We assume that everybody will be a mother—that's Garret Hardin's 'compulsory motherhood' concept. Hell, it's a privilege, it's not special enough. The contraceptive age affords us the opportunity to make motherhood really special...(p.181).

(My attitude on abortion) stems out of, I think, the same basic concern about the right (of children) to share the good life and all these things; children once born, have rights that we consistently deny them. I remember giving a talk (in which I said) that I thought one of my roles was to be an advocate for the fetus, and for the fetus's right not to be born...(p.182).

PSYCHOLOGICAL EFFECTS

The studies of women who have been denied abortions have produced conflicting results. While some of the research indicates that there are no harmful effects when women have been denied abortions, other studies indicate that there have been damaging results.

In a comprehensive review of almost 250 studies on the psychological effects of abortion, C. Everett Koop ("Effect of abortion", 1989) concluded that there was no definite evidence that abortions cause mental or physical problems in women. Although Koop wrote that many of the studies that were reviewed were methodologically flawed, the results did not support the conclusion that abortions contribute to psychological problems.

While some abortions could cause infertility or damage to the cervix, these physical problems could also develop in women who did not have abortions. Koop wrote that it would cost at least $10 million over the next five years to conduct an effective study of the psychological and physical effects of abortion.

In their book *Born Unwanted: Developmental Effects of Denied Abortion*, David, Dytrych, Matejcek, and Schuller (1988) carefully described a group of studies conducted in Sweden, Finland, and Czechoslovakia of children born to mothers who had been denied abortions. Although the authors reported the results of several studies, they emphasized the study that was conducted in Prague, Czechoslovakia because it was so well designed.

The Prague study is unique in that it is an on-going longitudinal study of children of women who had been twice denied abortion for the same pregnancy—on the first request and on appeal. The study used double-blind methods and matched each of the 110 boys and 110 girls who were born to women who had been denied abortions with children whose mothers had not requested abortions. The children were matched for sex, age, birth order, number of siblings, and grade in school; the mothers were matched for age, socioeconomic status, and for the husband's or partner's presence in the family. Extensive interviews and questionnaires were conducted with the children, the mothers, and teachers.

The Prague study found, along with the studies conducted in Sweden and Finland, that the children who were born unwanted were at risk of developing unhealthy personalities and of forming inadequate social relationships. While the researchers concluded that it was difficult to identify specific causal relationships, those children who were born unwanted did evidence more maladaptive behaviors and deprivation than the control group.

David et al. (1988) wrote:

> An unwanted pregnancy, operationally defined as actively rejected by the woman reasonably early in the gestation, leads, in the aggregate, to a social environment conducive to slightly deviant development in childhood and evolving into gradually worsening social difficulties and problems in adolescence and early adulthood, when compared to the social development of children born to women who accepted their pregnancy and did not request abortion (p.10).

In related research, the psychological risks of prenatal diagnostic testing were also examined. Hubbard (1982) felt that the risks of prenatal screening and diagnosis "are mainly social and psychological" (p.43). Prenatal diagnosis and its outcomes may be a source of considerable stress to parents and may interfere with the bonding process (Beeson, Douglas, & Lunsford, 1983).

Blumberg, Golbus, and Hanson (1975) studied 13 women and their families, in cases in which amniocentesis had been performed. Results showed a high incidence of depression in the mothers and fathers following abortion. They also found that a positive amniocentesis might be associated with the birth of a previously disabled child and thus the cycle of depression and guilt was resumed.

Marital difficulties were also reported. In another study, Farrant (1980) found that of the women who were waiting for the results of the amniocentesis, those with high AFP levels were more anxious than women with AFP levels that were within normal limits. Women with high AFP levels reported: "If they're inside you and you're worrying terrible it must affect them somehow"; "My husband's greatest worry was that the baby was perfectly normal but I would miscarry because I was so worried"; "I was worried about not eating—thinking I will miss the nutrition for the baby"; "I smoked a lot more and I was worried that it was not good for the baby" (Farrant, 1980 p.402).

SELECTIVE ABORTION

While some of the arguments concerning selective abortion are the same as the arguments concerning abortion, Silver (1981) stated that other arguments are germane to the issue of therapeutic abortion as well. While it is unknown how many fetuses are aborted after a positive result on a prenatal diagnostic test, there is evidence that shows that the incidence of abortions has increased for fetuses that have been diagnosed as having Down syndrome. Two studies (Hansen, 1978; Smith, Gardner, Steinhoff, Chung, & Palmore,

1980) examined the effect of abortion on the incidence of Down syndrome in Hawaii and New York state. Both of these studies concluded that the decrease in the incidence of Down syndrome was a direct result of the termination of a pregnancy through abortion and that selective abortion is an acceptable alternative to women who, as a result of prenatal diagnosis, learn that the fetus has Down syndrome.

Chapter 5 in this monograph discusses many of the ethical issues that arise when making treatment decisions for critically ill newborns. Although many of these issues are also pertinent here, the reader is encouraged to see Chapter 5 for an extended discussion of the following areas: personhood; sanctity of life; quality of life; provision of treatment; best interests; and the impact on society of the birth of a child with a handicap.

ARGUMENTS IN FAVOR OF
ABORTION

Proponents of selective abortion usually take the position that some benefit occurs because a fetus with a potential disability has been aborted. The benefits accrue to the fetus, the parents, the family, and society. For the fetus, one of the most frequently made arguments concerns the quality of life of the fetus after birth.

In somewhat paradoxical reasoning, it has been argued that some fetuses should not be born because many children who have medical problems such as spina bifida, hydrocephalus, and intestinal blockages are likely to face extensive surgery. Children born with Tay-Sachs disease will encounter a great deal of suffering before they eventually die (Lehr & Brown, 1984).

The legalization of abortion has greatly influenced patterns of marriage and childbearing (Cates, 1982). The use of prenatal diagnostic techniques and abortion after identification of a congenital disorder has benefited families who are at a known risk for genetic defects. The availability of these procedures has permitted couples to begin pregnancies they might not otherwise have undertaken or to continue pregnancies that they might have ended (Cates, 1982).

Aborting a fetus with a disorder may also benefit the parents by giving them the opportunity to begin a new pregnancy earlier than if the abnormal pregnancy had been allowed to come to term (Chervenak, Farley, Walters, Hobbins, & Mahoney, 1984).

Fletcher (1979) took a somewhat different position. While he accepted the abortion of a fetus in cases of severe disabilities, he did not accept euthanasia of newborns with disabilities. He wrote that there is a need to balance, what he termed the "growing right to life" (p.253) of the fetus with the needs of parents and society, which he felt outweigh fetal rights in abortion decisions:

...I do not hold that the fetus prior to viability is yet a fellow human being to whom wider social protection is due beyond the kind of educated care on the part of parents and physicians described above. Thus, if a severe defect is detected at this stage of development, one is morally justified to abort even though there will be much more emotional involvement in the second trimester since the fetus is felt to move. Parents who choose to abort at this stage act out of a desire to protect themselves, their family, and society from harm (Fletcher, 1979, p.249).

There can be societal benefits to terminating a pregnancy that is at risk. The medical costs associated with caring for the pregnant woman and the newborn are reduced considerably when a fetus is aborted. In addition, long-term costs relating to medical care for the child, education and training, and other expenses will not have to be undertaken if the child is not born. Chapter 5 includes additional discussion of these issues.

ARGUMENTS OPPOSING
SELECTIVE ABORTION

The discoverer of the chromosomal basis of Down syndrome, Lejune (Harris, 1975), argued that once an ovum is fertilized it is a human being. If the results of amniocentesis show the presence of a disorder in the fetus, the fetus should be protected because it has the same right to life as other fetuses that are free of disorders. Other geneticists argue that either the presence or the severity of a disorder is justification for abortion (Harris, 1975).

The strongest argument against selective abortion is made by opponents of abortion regardless of whether the fetus is normal or not. The main thrust of this argument is that abortion, for whatever reason, is wrong. The fetus, whether disabled or not, has a right to life and to quality care (Lehr & Brown, 1984).

When a fetus is aborted it may be thought of as a "product of conception," but if it is treated it is referred to as a "baby" and a "patient" (Callahan, 1986). For the treatment of disorders the fetus is viewed as having the same or almost the same rights as a patient, but if the disorders are untreatable any patient status is nullified by aborting the fetus. Is the treatable fetus viewed as superior, or more valued, than the nontreatable one?

Physicians have not been able to agree on their attitudes toward aborting fetuses after the diagnosis of a congenital disorder. Chervenak et al. (1984) wrote that only when two conditions are met can physicians morally justify terminating a pregnancy during the third trimester:

We argue that termination of pregnancy during the third trimester can also be morally justifiable (i.e., permissible) if two conditions are fulfilled: 1) the fetus is afflicted with a condition that is either a) incompatible with postnatal survival for more than a few weeks or b) characterized by the total or virtual absence of cognitive function; and 2) highly reliable diagnostic procedures

are available for determining prenatally that the fetus fulfills either condition
1a or 1b (p.501).

Anencephaly is the only condition that meets these two criteria. When
these authors considered other fetal disorders, such as renal agenesis, infan-
tile polycystic kidneys, Meckel's syndrome, trisomy 13, trisomy 18, alobar
holoprosencephaly, hyranencephaly, and Tay-Sachs disease, they concluded
that their criteria could not be adequately met (Chervenak et al., 1984).

Some ethicists have argued that selective abortion diminishes the life-
preserving role of the physician (Davis, 1981). In performing an abortion, the
physician is carrying out the wishes of the parents. Although parents may
cite therapeutic reasons for choosing an abortion, it has also been argued that
an abortion is never therapeutic for a fetus (Camenisch, 1984). Camenisch
(1984)—after posing the question "Abortion: for the fetus's own sake?"—
proceeded to write that:

> What is the value of existence per se, in the absence of health and normalcy?
> What is the difference, if any, between our responsibility for the things we
> do, the things we permit, the things we omit? Having bypassed these prob-
> lems, I can hardly conclude from the above thoughts that 'abortion for the
> fetus's own sake' is either a logical or a moral impossibility. I can only cite
> the difficulties I see in the use of such language and hope that those who
> continue to use it will be aware of these difficulties or will show the rest of
> us how they can be resolved (p.41).

Some physicians may be unwilling to perform abortions on fetuses that
have defects or disorders that are correctable (Callahan, 1986). The abortion
procedure may be easier on the woman if general anesthesia is used, but this
procedure may be more disturbing to physicians and nurses than if labor is
induced (although there may be little choice as to which procedure is used)
(Beeson, 1984).

The principle of beneficence holds that physicians do no harm and provide treatment whenever possible. But for some fetuses it can be argued that
it is difficult for physicians to determine whether their actions benefit or harm
the fetus. Some fetuses have disorders that prevent them from surviving more
than a few weeks after birth or conditions in which cognitive functioning is
nearly or completely absent. Delivery of these fetuses would result in early
death or a minimal existence (Chervenak et al., 1984).

A related argument is that errors can be made in prenatal diagnosis. Because the possibility of false-positive and false-negative errors exists, women
should not even consider prenatal diagnosis or, if they have made the mis-
take of undergoing prenatal diagnosis, they should not undergo an abortion.

While the results of some prenatal diagnostic techniques are available early
in the pregnancy, some results may take several weeks and cause the decision to have an abortion to be delayed. Thus, an additional dilemma of abortion

may be a live birth. Approximately 10% of second trimester abortions are performed on women who find out as a result of the amniocentesis that they are carrying a fetus with disorders (Kleiman, 1984). There is the likelihood of further injury to infants who are born after an attempted abortion and who already suffer from a chromosomal or metabolic disorder. Thus, advances in diagnostic medicine have contributed to a new problem—when abortion becomes birth (Kleiman, 1984). Some doctors may try to resuscitate the newborn; others do not consider it "viable" and choose not to treat it.

U.S. SUPREME COURT DECISIONS

The Supreme Court's decision in the *Roe v. Wade* case is viewed by pro-choice persons as protecting a woman's right to privacy and to giving a woman control over her own body. The ruling of the court was based on the argument that any state intrusion into a woman's relationship with her doctor and into a woman's decisions concerning reproduction violated her right to privacy. In effect, the *Roe v. Wade* decision ruled that women's rights superceded any rights the nonviable fetus may have.

In 1989, the U.S. Supreme Court, in an historic decision, *Webster, Attorney General of Missouri, et al. v. Reproductive Health Services et al.*, upheld three restrictions on abortion. As of this writing, the Court's ruling is limited to Missouri because no other state has enacted the same restrictions on abortion.

The Court ruled, in a 5 to 4 decision, that public hospitals or other facilities that are tax supported cannot be used to perform abortions, except to save the life of the mother, even when no public funds are used to perform the abortion. No public employee, including physicians, nurses, or other medical personnel, may perform or assist in the performance of an abortion except to save the mother's life. Finally, strict viability testing must be carried out on a fetus believed to be at least 20 weeks old before an abortion can be performed.

In effect, the *Webster* decision allows states to pass laws to restrict abortions. The *Webster* decision indicated that the U.S. Supreme Court does not consider abortion to be a fundamental right of women and ushered in a new era of debate on abortion (Greenhouse, 1989).

From a legal viewpoint, the decision in the *Webster* case increases the obligations to the fetus as the pregnancy progresses. The U.S. Supreme Court ruled in the *Webster* case that strict viability testing must be carried out on a fetus believed to be at least 20 weeks old before an abortion can be performed. Thus, even for a fetus believed to have a disorder, viability testing must be performed. These two decisions can actually be viewed as constitutional rulings that protect the fetus.

THE NEED FOR MORE DEBATE

Although there has already been considerable debate on this difficult topic, it seems that in a pluralistic society such as ours the debate must continue. It is especially urgent though, that concrete proposals and standards be established. The moving forces behind these issues are the lightning advance of technology, the rising costs associated with caring, educating, and training persons with disabilities, and the politicization of the issue of abortion. Research on the identification of disorders, both perinatally and prenatally, as well as intensive care for the tiniest and sickest newborns continues. Research and technology have far outpaced the development of ethical and legal standards.

Parents have an almost absolute right to decide whether to abort a fetus with a disability. Do parent's rights outweigh the rights of the fetus to be born? A review of the court cases relating to abortion have affirmed the parent's rights. The growing legal rights of the fetus must be clarified through legislative action and court review.

The improvement in the quality of life for persons with severe disabilities has been documented. These improvements should be shared with parents and professionals in medicine, law, social welfare, and education so that these individuals understand that persons who are disabled can have a quality life.

Society has been reluctant to question the abortion of fetuses that are disabled or have the potential of being disabled. Fetuses with Down syndrome and other handicaps may be aborted for any "normal" reason, or because of some disabling condition. The issue of aborting a fetus 'for its own good' and for the welfare of the family and society must be raised. How should we respond to the diagnosis of a fetus with chromosomal and metabolic disorders?

A child that is disabled may be seen as a person who need not have lived, "if only someone had gotten to him in time. . .The idea of the 'unwanted because abnormal child' may become a self-fulfilling prophecy, whose consequences may be worse than those of the abnormality itself" (Harris, 1975, p.79). Negative eugenic policies could encourage the prevention and elimination of persons who have undesirable genes (Harris, 1975) and could lead to mandatory genetic screening of all parents and mandatory abortion of fetuses with defects.

Few parent or professional organizations have examined the consequences of selectively aborting fetuses after the diagnosis of fetal damage. Although many of these organizations actively support research on the identification and treatment of congenital disorders, none have supported selective abortion as a way of preventing cognitive and physical disabilities (Wilke, cited in Smith, 1981).

The abortion of a fetus that has been diagnosed as having a chromosomal or metabolic disorder devalues children and adults who are disabled. A person who is healthy and normal is evaluated by society as better. But who decides what is healthy and normal?

REFERENCES

Abortion: Women speak out, an exclusive poll. (1981, November). *Life*, pp.45-54.

Beeson, D. (1984). Technological rhythms in pregnancy: The case of prenatal diagnosis by amniocentesis. In T. Duster & K. Garrett (Eds.), *Biological rhythms and social relations* (pp.145-181). Norwood, NJ: Ablex.

Beeson, D., Douglas, R., & Lunsford, T. F. (1983). Prenatal diagnosis of fetal disorders. Part II: Issues and implications. *Birth, 10,* 233-241.

Blumberg, B. D., Golbus, M. S., & Hanson, K. H. (1975). The psychological sequalae of abortion performed for a genetic indication. *American Journal of Obstetrics and Gynecology, 122,* 799-808.

Callahan, D. (1986). How technology is reframing the abortion debate. *The Hastings Center Report, 16,* 33-42.

Camenisch, P. (1984). Abortion: for the fetus's own sake? *The Hastings Center Report,* April.

Cates, Jr., W. (1982). Legal abortion: The public health record. *Science, 215,* 1586-1590.

Chervenak, F. A., Farley, M. A., Walters, L., Hobbins, J. C., & Mahoney, M. J. (1984). When is termination of pregnancy during the third trimester morally justifiable? *The New England Journal of Medicine, 310,* 501-504.

Cohen, L. (1986). Selective abortion and the diagnosis of fetal damage: Issues and concerns. *The Journal of the Association for Persons with Severe Handicaps, 11,* 188-195.

David, H. P., Dytrych, Z., Matejeck, Z., & Schuller, V. (1988). *Born unwanted: Developmental effects of denied abortion.* New York: Springer.

Davis, J.G. (1981). Ethical issues arising from prenatal diagnosis. *Mental Retardation, 19* (1), 12-15.

Dionne, Jr., E. J. (1989, April 26). Poll on abortion finds the nation is sharply divided. *The New York Times,* pp.1, 25.

Effect of abortion on women is discounted. (1989, January 10). *The New York Times,* p.A19.

Farrant, W. (1980). Stress after amniocentesis for high serum alpha-fetoprotein concentrations. *British Medical Journal, 9,* 402.

Fletcher, J. (1979). Prenatal diagnosis, selective abortion and the ethics of withholding treatment from the defective newborn. In A. Capron, M. Loppe, R.F. Murray, T. Powledge, S. Twiss, & D. Bergsma (Eds.), *Abortion: Moral and Legal Perspectives.* Amherst: The University of Massachusetts Press.

Greenhouse, L. (1989, July 4). Supreme Court, 5-4. narrowing *Roe v. Wade,* upholds sharp state limits on abortions. *The New York Times,* pp.1, 10.

Hansen, H. (1978). Decline of Down's Syndrome after abortion reform in New York state. *American Journal of Mental Deficiency, 83,* 185-188.

Harris, H. (1975). *Prenatal Diagnosis and Selective Abortion.* Cambridge: Harvard University Press.

Hellegers, A. E. (1978). Medical context of abortion. In W. T. Reich (Ed.), *Encyclopedia of Bioethics,* Vol. 1 (pp.1-5). New York: Free Press.

Henry, N. F., & Harvey, M. E. (1982). Social, spatial, and political determinants of U. S. abortion rates. *Social Science and Medicine, 16,* 987-996.

Hubbard, R. (1982). Some practical and ethical constraints on genetic decisions about childbearing. In D. Teichler-Zallen & C. D. Clements (Eds.), *Science and Morality: New Directions in Bioethics.* Lexington, MA: Lexington Books.

Kleiman, D. (1984, February 15). When abortion becomes birth: A dilemma of medical ethics shaken by new advances. *The New York Times,* p.B1.

Kolata, G. (1988a, June 2). Study finds rate of abortion is high among U.S. women. *The New York Times,* p.A22.

Kolata, G. (1988b, October 6). Studies find abortion rate staying constant. *The New York Times,* A24.

Lehr, D., & Brown, F. (1984). Perspectives on severely multiply handicapped. In E. Meyer (Ed.), *Mental Retardation: Topics of Today—Issues of Tomorrow,* (pp.41-65). Reston, VA: Council for Exceptional Children.

Luker, K. (1984a). *Abortion and the Politics of Motherhood,* (pp.158-191). Los Angeles: University of California Press.

Luker, K. (1984b). Abortion and the meaning of life. In S. Callahan & D. Callahan (Eds.), *Abortion Understanding Differences* (pp.25-45). New York: Plenum Press.

McLoughlin, M. (1988, October 3). America's new civil war. *U.S. News & World Report, 105,* 22-31.

Reich, W. T. (Ed.) (1978). *Encyclopedia of Bioethics,* Vol. 1. New York: Free Press.

Silver, T. (1981). Amniocentesis and selective abortion. *Pediatric Annals, 10,* 397-400.

Smith, J. D. (1981). Down's Syndrome, amniocentesis, and abortion: Prevention or elimination? *Mental Retardation, 19* (1), 8-11.

Smith, R. G., Gardner, R. W., Steinhoff, P., Chung, C. S., & Palmore, J. A. (1980). The effect of induced abortion on the incidence of Down's syndrome in Hawaii. *Family Planning Perspectives, 12,* 201-205.

Tietze, C. (1984). The public health effects of legal abortion in the United States. *Family Planning Perspectives, 16,* 26-28.

Warren, M. (1978). On the moral and legal status of abortion. In T.L. Beauchamp & L. Walters (Eds.), *Contemporary Issues in Bioethics.* Encino, CA: Dickenson.

Webster, Attorney General of Missouri, et al. v. Reproductive Health Services et al., No. 88-605, slip op. (U.S., July 3, 1989).

Chapter 4

The Devaluing of Infants and Children with Disabilities

How a society values the health, safety and welfare of its members is reflected in how and to what extent the state protects its citizens through law (Damme, 1978, p.1).

...I have given suck, and know How tender 'tis to love the babe that milks me: I would, while it was smiling in my face, Have pluck'd my nipple from his boneless gums, And dashed the brains out, had I so sworn as you Have done to this (Lady Macbeth, Macbeth, Act I, Scene 7).

Persons with disabilities have been the targets of discriminatory attitudes and behaviors almost since the beginning of time. Having a disability has meant that individuals have been devalued. At various times, persons with disabilities could be disposed of, given inadequate medical care, denied education, refused meaningful employment, isolated, segregated, and ignored. Although, in recent years, many of these discriminatory attitudes and behaviors have receded, there is evidence that they still exist.

Two of the ways that infants and children with disabilities have been and continue to be discriminated against are by deliberately killing them and by providing inadequate medical care. While these two issues have been well documented and publicized, it is important to review them.

Although we condemn its practice, the killing of infants and children with disabilities continues to be committed world wide, both overtly and covertly, in primitive, industrialized and post-industrialized societies. Infanticide, which is the willful killing of a child under one year of age, has taken many forms. Children have been poisoned, strangled, suffocated, starved, abandoned, thrown into rivers, burned to death, put in large jars, beaten to death, and killed with lethal weapons (Montag & Montag, 1979; Langer, 1974).

Euthanasia of infants with disabilities, which is the termination of the life of the infant in order to prevent further suffering when there is no hope of survival, is different from infanticide in that infanticide does not have the connotation of preventing suffering. The ethical issues associated with the euthanasia of infants with disabilities are discussed in Chapter 5.

Infanticide has varied over time and in different societies. It has been frequently encouraged; only rarely have penalties been given. During certain periods of history, infanticide was practiced almost relentlessly; during other times, the practice subsided. Although prohibited by law in many countries, it continues for a variety of reasons.

Paralleling the attitudes of society to children in general, Scheerenberger (1983) pointed out that the treatment of persons with mental retardation has also varied. Some societies and cultures have been compassionate and just, while others have acted very harshly. In particular, the followers of Zoroaster, Buddha, Confucius, Jesus, and Mohammed were urged to follow humanitarian ideals. Scheerenberger wrote that "Each of these religious leaders expressed precepts that in no manner would bring harm to mentally retarded persons or others with afflictions" (Scheerenberger, 1983, p.22).

Ancient cultures were superstitious and believed that deformities were portents of good or evil. The supernatural origin of defects has been traced to North Africa and has been associated with witches and demons (Fletcher, 1974). The belief then spread to Greece where Plato advocated the practice of infanticide in order to rid society of deformed people (Montag & Montag, 1979).

From there, the practice of infanticide spread to Rome. Myth relates that Rome was founded by Romulus and Remus, two children who were abandoned (Langer, 1974). Although, according to the legend, Romulus proclaimed that all infants who were not handicapped or deformed should be kept alive (Garrison, 1965), the Romans practiced infanticide on a regular basis and were unconerned about the medical care of newborns who were disabled. Children who were first born males, without any disabilities, were the most likely to survive (Weir, 1984). The Romans believed that it was wise to kill infants who were disabled and that only the fittest should be allowed to live (Sumner, 1906).

The parents of newborns who were born disabled were frequently tortured and killed. Maternal fright was an explanation that was frequently offered for the birth of a child with a disability. European, Middle Eastern, Eskimo, and African cultures believed that sudden fright and the mental outlook of the mother could result in the birth of a child with a disability (Fletcher, 1974). For example, being frightened by a rabbit could result in a harelip.

A prevalent attitude toward children with disabilities during the Middle Ages and continuing until the Enlightenment was that a child with a disability was a changeling. A changeling was the child of demons who lived under the earth and envied the beauty of humans and their immortal soul. Because of this, they stole human children and exchanged them for their own (Haffter, 1968).

Parents were encouraged to kill these changelings. Fairy tales portrayed the changeling as peculiar in appearance. The body was out of proportion; it had a large head with an ugly, wrinkled face. According to legend, it was not a child at all but an "age-old creature" (Haffter, 1968, p.56). It was believed that the child with the disability had been substituted shortly after the birth of the real child and was possessed by demons.

Various methods were used to get rid of the changeling and get the real child back. A common method was that of tricking it to laugh or talk. If that did not work, the changeling was cruelly treated so that the real parents would feel sorry for it and come and take it away:

> One should hold it over boiling water and threaten to plunge it in. The oven should be heated with nine different kinds of wood and the child placed on the shovel as if it was intended to thrust it into the fire. The child should be placed on the red-hot shovel, pressed into red-hot ashes, laid on a red-hot grid, shots should be fired over it, it should be fed on leather and red-hot iron, it should be given poison to drink (Haffter, 1968, p.57).

The idea that a child who was disabled was subhuman has continued. Children with disabilities have been portrayed as being descended from primitive peoples. In Switzerland, "mongoloid" features were attributed to the Huns who invaded Europe during the 5th century (Haffter, 1968). Haffter (1968) believes that Langdon Down's "Ethnic Classification of Idiots" provided a scientific rationale for the belief that children who were disabled were descended from primitive races and were a throwback to earlier times.

The church provided a religious rationale for the idea of a changeling: that the changeling was actually a form of the devil. If somehow the child who was handicapped survived infancy, other penalties awaited the child including segregation, banishment, oppression, and cruelty.

Societies have permitted the practice of infanticide for many reasons including population control, illegitimacy, lack of ability to care for infants, superstition, sacrifice, reduction of the number of unproductive individuals, preference for male children, the physical deformities of children, greed, power, post partum depression, and, protection of the mother (Montag & Montag, 1979). Other reasons include eugenics, poverty, economics, and the belief in many societies that infants with disabilities are somehow inferior, less desirable, and expendable.

A frequent explanation that was offered for killing newborns with disabilities is that it was economically expedient. If a child was thought to be unproductive and unable to contribute to the maintenance of the family, because of some deformity, it could be killed.

Lack of financial resources continues to be an argument advocated by some today. Children with disabilities may require extensive medical care, and for most families the costs of this care can be financially crippling. This is a complex issue for families and for society as a whole; a discussion of the financial, emotional, and physical burdens that many families of children with disabilities carry will follow later in this book.

In recent times, the most horrific practice of the killing of children with handicaps occurred under the Nazis. Wolfensberger (1981) and others have discussed the systematic program of killing of children who were disabled. Although the origins of this Nazi policy can be traced to early in the 20th century, Hitler's authorization for the program came in 1939.

It has been estimated that as many as 1,000,000 persons (including children and adults) were systematically put to death because they were disabled. Wolfensberger wrote that the Nazis were so successful that when he visited an institution in Germany for persons with mental retardation, there were very few adult residents. Six methods of killing were employed including gassing, poisoning, injections, starvation, withholding care, and exposure.

Lifton (1986), in his book, *The Nazi Doctors,* has meticulously documented the participation of physicians in Nazi Germany in the killing of children with handicaps and in the extermination of millions of people. Around 1941, mass killing began in Nazi Germany. Up until that time, the murder of children had been supposedly based on eugenic and scientific reasons. Any child who was disabled could be identified and the child's future left to the prerogative of individual physicians. Frequent methods of killing were through the use of fatal injections, oral medication, and starvation.

Children were also used for medical experimentation. Mengele, the infamous Nazi doctor, was maniacal in his pursuit of children and adults who were suitable subjects for his research. At Auschwitz, he established special areas set aside for research on twins, dwarfs, and children with abnormalities. After studying his subjects, he might kill them himself or order that they be killed. Finally, Mengele would painstakingly examine and dissect their corpses.

In the United States, there is no federal law that prohibits infanticide. Persons who commit infanticide are usually prosecuted under state laws that prohibit homicide. Although infanticide is the killing of a human being, it has been viewed as different from homicide, and the penalties for infanticide, if any are invoked, are not as great as the penalties given for homicide (Damme, 1978). Weir (1984) pointed out that in the U.S. the condemnation of infanticide has varied:

> The reasons for the current uncertainty of punishment in the United States are several: enormous weight is given to parental autonomy, importance is placed on medical discretion when infant deaths occur in clinical settings, infants (especially neonates) are often believed to have a lesser legal status than do older children and adults, no laws exist that specifically proscribe infanticide, and parents (usually mothers) tried for child homicide are often acquitted for reasons of temporary insanity (p.5).

MEDICAL CARE AND TREATMENT

Wolfensberger (1989), who does not distinguish between infanticide and euthanasia, wrote that there are policies now in place that sanction the euthanasia of people with mental retardation:

> For instance, with the administration of liquids and nourishment being

euphemistically redefined as "medical treatment," and with the legalization of the withholding of such treatments from debilitated people (who may be neither comatose nor "dying," as if that mattered), sick retarded people are certainly one of the groups who are being deprived of life (p.63).

Handicapism, a set of beliefs that perpetuate the unequal treatment of people because of apparent or assumed behavioral, mental, or physical differences, is pervasive in the medical treatment of children who are born with a disability. Different criteria are used when making medical care decisions about persons with and without disabilities. "The arguments of those who think there should be different criteria for a decision to treat a child with a potentially severe disability reveal some of our society's most deeply seated prejudices regarding disabled people" (Bogdan & Knoll, 1988, p.471).

Many organizations that advocate on behalf of people with disabilities have issued resolutions opposing treatment decisions based on whether the infant has a disability, regardless of the severity of the disability. Representative of these are the resolutions issued by the American Association on Mental Retardation, The Association for Persons with Severe Handicaps, and the Council for Exceptional Children, Division on Mental Retardation. The Association for Persons with Severe Handicaps (TASH) adopted a resolution in 1983 that to end the life of an infant with severe disabilities either directly or by withholding food or treatment is discriminatory. The Council for Exceptional Children, Division on Mental Retardation issued a similar statement in 1988.

The following statement issued by the American Association on Mental Retardation and signed by the American Academy of Pediatrics, the American Association of University Affiliated Programs for the Developmentally Disabled, the American Coalition of Citizens with Disabilities, the Association for Retarded Citizens, the Down Syndrome Congress, the National Association of Children's Hospitals and Related Institutions, the Spina Bifida Association of America, and the Association for the Severely Handicapped, affirmed that persons with disabilities are entitled to the same rights as all other members of our society:

Principles of Treatment of Disabled Infants

Discrimination of any type against any individual with a disability/disabilities regardless of the nature or severity of the disability is morally and legally indefensible. Throughout their lives, all disabled individuals have the same rights as other citizens, including access to such major society activities as health care, education and employment. These rights for all disabled persons must be recognized at birth.

Medical Care

When medical care is clearly beneficial, it should always be provided. When appropriate medical care is not available, arrangements should be made to transfer the infant to an appropriate medical facility. Consideration such as anticipated or actual limited potential of an individual and present or future lack of available community resources are irrelevant and must not determine the decisions concerning medical care. The individual's medical condition should be the sole focus of the decision. These are very strict standards.

It is ethically and legally justified to withhold medical or surgical procedures which are clearly futile and will only prolong the act of dying. However, supportive care should be provided including sustenance as medically indicated and relief of pain and suffering. The needs of the dying person should be respected. The family should also be supported in their grieving.

In cases where it is uncertain whether medical treatment will be beneficial, a person's disability must not be the basis for a decision to withhold treatment. At all times during the process when decisions are being made about the benefit or futility of medical treatment, the person should be cared for in the medically most appropriate ways. When doubt exists at any time about whether to treat, a presumption always should be made in favor of treatment (Berkowitz, 1983, p.263).

In 1989, the U.S. Commission on Civil Rights issued the report *Medical Discrimination Against Children with Disabilities*, which concluded that there is "no doubt that newborn children have been denied food, water, and medical treatment solely because they are, or are perceived to be, disabled" (p.3). Based on the testimony of experts and anecdotal reports, the Commission wrote that it is likely that the denial of lifesaving treatment to children with disabilities is "widespread" (p.148) and discriminatory.

Despite documentation in numerous journal articles and by the media of the withholding of food and medical care to infants with handicaps, the devaluing continues. It is perplexing that the devaluing of infants and children with handicaps occurs at a time when the rights of people with disabilities are expanding (Rosenblum & Budde, 1982). Federal mandates protect the civil rights of people with disabilities as well as their right to education and training, yet the care and protection of infants with disabilities remains a deeply troubling area of concern.

REFERENCES

Berkowitz, A. (1983). National news. *Mental Retardation, 21,* 263-264.

Bogdan, R., & Knoll, J. (1988). The sociology of disability. In E. L. Meyen & T. M. Skrtic (Eds.), *Exceptional children and youth* (3rd ed.), Denver: Love Publishing.

Damme, C. (1978). Infanticide: The worth of an infant under law. *Medical History, 22,* 1-24.

Fletcher, J. C. (1974). Attitudes toward defective newborns. *The Hastings Center Studies, 2,* 21-32.

Garrison, F. H. (1965). History of pediatrics. In A. F. Abt, & F. H. Garrison (Eds.). *History of Pediatrics* (pp.1-170). Philadelphia: W. B. Saunders.

Haffter, C. (1968). The changeling: History and psychodynamics of attitudes to handicapped children in European folklore. *Journal of the History of the Behavioral Sciences, 4,* 55-61.

Langer, W. L. (1974). Infanticide: A historical survey. *History of Childhood Quarterly, 1,* 353-365.

Lifton, R. J. (1986). *The Nazi Doctors*. New York: Basic Books.

Montag, B. A., & Montag, T. W. (1979). Infanticide a historical perspective. *Minnesota Medicine, 62,* 368-372.

Rosenblum, V. G., & Budde, M. L. (1982). Historical and cultural considerations of infanticide. In D. J. Horan & M. Delahoyde (Eds.). *Infanticide and the Handicapped Newborn* (pp.1-16). Provo, UT: Brigham Young University.

Scheerenberger, R. C. (1983). *A history of mental retardation*. Baltimore: Paul H. Brookes.

Sumner, W. G. (1906). *Folkways*. Boston: Ginn and Company.

U.S. Commission on Civil Rights (1989). Medical discrimination against children with disabilities. Washington, DC: U.S. Commission on Civil Rights.

Weir, R. (1984). *Selective Nontreatment of Handicapped Newborns*. New York: Oxford University Press.

Wolfensberger, W. (1981). The extermination of handicapped people in World War II Germany. *Mental Retardation, 19,* 1-17.

Wolfensberger, W. (1989). The killing thought in the eugenic era and today: A commentary on Hollander's essay. *Mental Retardation, 27,* 63-65.

Chapter 5

Newborns with Severe Disabilities: Ethical Issues

During the next seventeen days Christopher's condition remained poor. He had poor reflexes, poor muscle tone, and frequent convulsions. At this time his long-term outlook was thought to include severe mental retardation, possible continuing uncontrollable convulsions, possible deafness, possible blindness, possible cerebral palsy, and motor defects that might be extensive enough to make him a quadriplegic. Brain damage was believed to be generalized and extensive and was thought to involve the cortex (Bridge & Bridge, 1981, p.17).

This excerpt, from an article by Christopher Bridge's parents in which they related their experiences in making treatment decisions for their son, highlights the life-threatening circumstances that parents and health care providers face when an infant is born with a severely disabling condition. Christopher's parents agonized over his treatment for 75 days, until his death from cardiac arrest and oxygen deprivation (Bridge & Bridge, 1981).

The infants that are the focus of this chapter are the sickest, most critically ill newborns found in intensive care nurseries. Frequently, they are premature and have a low birthweight (less than 1500 grams); others are born with a congenital disorder. Many come into this world with a variety of life-threatening medical problems including hyaline membrane disease, which is caused by immature lung development, asphyxia, which is lack of oxygen, hypothermia, hypoglycemia, infections, jaundice, congenital problems, cardiac disease (McCormick, 1985), and irregular brain development.

The number of newborns born with severely disabling conditions is large. The population of the world has been estimated to increase by approximately 82 million persons a year. At this rate, approximately 20,000 children who have some disability are born every day. Estimates of the percent of all babies born alive who may have some type of birth defect range from 3-15% (Kevles, 1985; Lyon, 1985). In addition, there has been a drastic increase in the number of babies born with disabilities whose mothers abused drugs and/or alcohol.

Although the incidence of each type of birth disorder is low, when the various types of disabling conditions are combined, total incidence is high (Lyon, 1985). For example, Down syndrome, occurs 8.5 times in every 10,000 live births; hydrocephalus without spina bifida, happens 4.8 times out of every 10,000 live births; microcephaly strikes 2.5 times out of every 10,000 live

53

births; trachea-esophageal anomalies occur 2.1 times in every 10,000 live births; and ventricular septal defects happen 17.1 times in every 10,000 live births (U.S. Commission on Civil Rights, 1989).

Twenty to thirty percent of all children who are admitted to hospitals have a congenital disorder (Kevles, 1985). A high percentage of the deaths of children younger than one year of age are attributed to congenital conditions. As of 1983 these included: 62% of infants born with spina bifida; 59% of infants born with hydrocephalus; 86% of infants born with anencephaly; and 36% of all infants born with microcephaly. Sixty-two percent of all children younger than one year who were born with cardiovascular problems died and 47% of infants born with gastrointestinal defects died (U.S. Commission on Civil Rights, 1989). Although the death of an infant may be attributed to one of these conditions, it is unknown to what extent these children died because they were denied medical treatment.

There are many issues that surround the birth of a newborn with a severely disabling condition, including social, economic, psychological, legal, and ethical issues. This chapter will explore some of the ethical issues that arise when making treatment decisions for critically ill newborns, as well as the implications for society of caring for these infants. In examining each of the issues, the views of representative writers are presented.

EUTHANASIA

Euthanasia is the intentional termination of the life of a person in order to prevent further suffering. In the United States, the practice of euthanasia is illegal (Angell, 1988). During the past few years, the debate over whether it is permissible to end the life of a critically ill infant has intensified. Should the life of an individual be ended, thereby beginning "a step down a slippery slope leading to a widespread disregard for the value of human life," or should there be "an opportunity to deal more humanely and rationally with prolonged meaningless suffering" (Angell, 1988, p.1348)?

While this debate continues it seems that some physicians, ethicists, and laypersons agree that it is permissible to practice euthanasia under certain circumstances and that in fact, despite the legal prohibitions, euthanasia is currently being practiced (Duff & Campbell (1973; 1976).

Another debate has emerged over whether euthanasia should be practiced actively or passively. Although there is a fine line between the two, *passive euthanasia* refers to withholding or withdrawing of medical treatment or sustenance in order to allow a patient to die, while *active euthanasia* indicates using direct means, such as a lethal injection, to assist a patient in dying (Rachels, 1975).

The American Medical Association, in a statement issued in 1973, affirmed that the intentional killing of another person is contrary to the policies of that organization. But the statement went on to say that the decision to halt the use of extraordinary means to prolong life when there is no hope of recovery can be made by the physician, the patient, and the family (Rachels, 1975).

The distinction that is made between active and passive euthanasia is that the latter presumes that a patient is allowed to die, while the former means that the patient is assisted in dying. For a patient who has endured agonized suffering, who is expected to die within a few days, and who no longer wants to live, is it merciful to withhold treatment while at the same time making the patient as comfortable as possible? Is it kinder to give a lethal injection in order to end the suffering? Is it more humane to stand by and watch the person continue to suffer or is it more humane to assist the person in dying (Rachels, 1975)?

PERSONHOOD

Although the Constitution of the United States guarantees equal protection of the law to all persons, it does not define what a *person* is. Ethicists and philosophers have offered various arguments on who a person is and how personhood should be defined. If personhood can be established, it is reasoned, then it can be determined if and when fetuses can be aborted and newborns who are critically ill can be allowed to die without any moral prohibitions.

Joseph Fletcher (1978) has developed criteria of personhood which include minimal intelligence (IQ above 20), self-awareness, self-control, a sense of time, a sense of control of existence, curiosity, change and changeability, balance of rationality and feeling, idiosyncrasy, and neocortical function. Just how many of these criteria are enough to be able to label a human a person, and how these criteria are to be determined and evaluated is unclear.

According to Fletcher, the central question is not whether an infant is a person or not, but rather whether a person's life can be ended ethically. The emphasis is placed on the value of a human life rather than on keeping someone alive. Value must be established on the well-being of the individual through helping the person attain happiness or by helping to limit suffering. We are obliged to ensure well-being and this may mean that infanticide can be practiced. "If one's standard of the good is human well-being, and one's duty or obligation is to seek to increase it wherever possible, with a consequent willingness to save lives sometimes and end them sometimes, then it will follow that infanticide is acceptable (sometimes)" (Fletcher, 1978, pp.20-21).

Kluge (1980), in a discussion of the criteria for brain death, wrote that although an individual's brain may have ceased to function, a person may still be considered to be alive when the traditional criteria of presence of heartbeat and respiration are used. Writing that conscious awareness is a human capability, Kluge argued that heartbeat and respiration indicate only that the individual is a member of the species *Homo sapiens*, a biological entity, but not necessarily a person. By making a distinction between a person, a constructive person, and a human being, Kluge proposed that certain neonates, for whom there is no hope of survival, could be allowed to die.

The category of *person* includes the categories *natural person* and *constructive person.* A natural person is a human being who is capable of conscious awareness or has a cerebrum that is structurally and neurologically similar to that of a normal adult human being. A constructive person is any association of persons able to act as a social intermediary similar to a natural person. A *human* is any living biological being that is a part of the species *Homo sapiens* (Kluge, 1980).

Building on these distinctions, Kluge (1980) then argued that in instances in which "the whole range of brain damage cases, which otherwise would be (and currently are) problematic (p.253), could be resolved using the following criteria:

1. A human being becomes a natural person within the meaning of this (proposed) Act when it has acquired the present functional capability for conscious awareness, whether or not
   a. it has proceeded from its place of gestation or
   b. it has actually realized this capability in any observable manner.
2. A human being ceases to be a natural person when the neurological basis of his present functional capability for conscious awareness is irreparably destroyed or damaged beyond functional recovery within the limits of personhood as set out in section 2 above (pp.253-254).

Using these criteria, Kluge continued, would prevent the unnecessary prolongation of life of infants for whom there was no hope of survival and would relieve health care providers from being in conflict with current laws that prohibit homicide, child abuse, and neglect.

Another philosopher who distinguished between infants and persons is Michael Tooley. In the book, *Abortion and Infanticide,* Tooley (1983) wrote that:

> an entity cannot be a person unless it possesses, or has previously possessed, the capacity for thought. And the psychological and neurological evidence makes it most unlikely that humans, in the first few weeks after birth, possess this capacity (p.421).

Certain conditions must exist in order to make a being a person and these conditions include "the possession, either now or at some time in the past, of a sense of time, of a concept of continuing subject of mental states, and of a capacity for thought episodes" (Tooley, 1983, pp.419-420). Infants are not persons because they do not possess self-consciousness, sense of the future, or hopes about the future. Those infants who have suffered brain damage are not even potential persons, and for these, the traditional principles of morality do not apply and infanticide does not have to be rejected.

Tooley (1979) also reasoned that the quality of life for infants who are severely disabled is poor. Some infants may be so severely impaired that they are not aware of themselves or of others around them. He concluded that it is permissible to practice euthanasia or infanticide.

Questioning two of the consequences of the practice of infanticide, Tooley wrote that one of these, the so-called "slippery slope consequence," that acceptance of infanticide will lead to a lessening of the respect for the lives of other humans— rests on the assumption that being a member of the species *Homo sapiens* makes it wrong to kill other humans.

But this assumption is faulty because the moral prohibitions against killing do not contain any references to being a member of a particular species. The second consequence, that acceptance of infanticide will lead to a diminishment of parental feeling, Tooley also dismissed; parents who do not destroy their children (whom they would have liked to destroy) will not love them as much as other children and will treat them harshly.

Tooley summarized his position:

> In conclusion, then, there do not appear to be strong consequentialist grounds for rejecting infanticide. For while it is not implausible to think that there may be some negative consequences associated with acceptance of infanticide, for some people, there would also seem to be excellent reason (sic) for thinking that these effects will be short-term ones, and that they will be significantly outweighed by the positive consequences that will flow from the adoption of sound moral principles in this area (Tooley, 1983, pp.415-416).

The argument that infants are not persons has been rebutted by Taub (1982), Robertson (1975), and English (1975). Taub, in a discussion of the criteria for personhood, wrote that if the criteria for personhood were strictly applied, many functioning adults would be eliminated. Robertson reasoned that every infant is human and has a right to exist; since the determination of the severity of mental retardation usually cannot be made until the child is older, it is wrong to condemn infants who may be disabled to death.

The features of typical persons were described by English (1975):

> Within our concept of a person we include, first, certain biological factors: descended from humans, having a certain genetic make-up, having a head, hands, arms, eyes, capable of locomotion, breathing, eating, sleeping. There are psychological factors: sentience, perception, having a concept of self and of one's own interests and desires, the ability to use tools, the ability to use language or symbol systems, the ability to joke, to be angry, to doubt. There are rationality factors: the ability to reason and draw conclusions, the ability to generalize and to learn from past experience, the ability to sacrifice present interests for greater gains in the future. There are social factors: the ability to work in groups and respond to peer pressures, the ability to recognize and consider as valuable the interests of others, seeing oneself as one among "other minds," the ability to sympathize, encourage, love, the ability to work with others for mutual advantage. Then there are legal factors: being subject to the law and protected by it, having the ability to sue and enter contracts,

being counted in the census, having a name and citizenship, the ability to own property, inherit, and so forth (pp.419-420).

While this very long list of features of a typical person has been enumerated, English reasoned that each of these features could be rebutted. She wrote, "There is no single core of necessary and sufficient features which we can draw upon with the assurance that they constitute what really make a person; there are only features that are more or less typical" (English, 1975, p.420).

SANCTITY OF LIFE

The position that life is sacred and that sanctity of life is the most important consideration when deciding whether to treat newborns with disabilities is taken by several authors. Human life is considered intrinsically valuable by these authors, and any form of life is preferable to death. This viewpoint was represented by Jakobovits (1978), by Devlin and Magrab (1981), and by Gustafson (1973).

In a chapter titled "Jewish Views of Life," Jakobovits (1978) wrote that unless infants are expected to die, no matter how severely disabled they are, treatment must be provided. Life has infinite worth and all life is "equally valuable and inviolable" (Jakobovits, 1978, p.27).

Because the lives of all persons, even persons who are severely disabled, are cherished, the practice of euthanasia is condemned in the same way that infanticide is denounced. Writing that the relief of pain and suffering cannot be used as a reason to allow infants to die, Jakobovits urged society to provide economic, institutional, and social relief to alleviate pain and suffering. The euthanasia of any person who is judged to be inferior is not tolerated because, "Once a single brick is removed from the dam protecting the sanctity of all life, the entire dam is liable to collapse and every life is at risk" (Jakobovits, 1978, p.28).

This position was also supported by Devlin and Magrab (1981), who believed that every infant is a person and is entitled to the right to the protection of life. This right is inviolable and universal and all treatment decisions should be based on it. Although an infant is severely disabled, this right should not be diminished. The only circumstances that would permit violating this right to life and the withholding of care is when maintaining life becomes an agonized and unnecessarily prolonged process of dying.

The well-being of family members should not be a concern, according to Devlin and Magrab. Medical costs, as well as the psychological impact of caring for a child with severe disabilities, should not be considered when making treatment decisions. By advocating adherence to the fundamental principle of right-to-life, they believed that they were advancing a justification for the provision of social services to families and children with handicaps.

In an analysis of the Johns Hopkins baby who was born with Down syndrome and an intestinal blockage and who was allowed to die of starvation, Gustafson (1973) took a position similar to that of Devlin and Magrab. He wrote that there is a moral obligation to keep infants alive and that the basic rights of a person should not be compromised "by any given person's intelligence or capacities for productivity, potential consequences of the sort that burden others" (Gustafson, 1973, p.552).

Infants with disabilities are humans and because of this they should be intrinsically valued. Once a baby is born, the parents and the medical professionals are obligated to care for it and to maintain its life, regardless of other considerations. Actions should always be taken to sustain life through ordinary methods. The needs of other individuals should not be used as a rationale for withholding care; this will only serve to nullify the rights of the infant.

Is the position that life is sacrosanct and inviolable tenable? This concept is culturally based and varies with different ethnic groups and religious beliefs. Besides the conviction that infants are truly persons, other considerations include the quality of life of persons with severe disabilities, parental and family interests, and the best interests of the child.

QUALITY OF LIFE

Peter Singer (1979; 1983) believed that the quality of life is an important consideration when making treatment decisions about infants who are critically ill or who are handicapped. Criticizing the sanctity of life position, he wrote:

> If we can put aside the obsolete and erroneous notion of the sanctity of all human life, we may start to look at human life as it really is: at the quality of life that each human being has or can achieve. Then it will be possible to approach these difficult questions of life and death with the ethical sensitivity that each case demands. . . .(Singer, 1983, p.129).

According to Singer, ethical decisions can no longer be based on the belief that human beings have been specially created, formed in the image of God, and have an immortal soul. Comparing a hypothetical infant who is severely disabled with nonhuman animals, he concluded that the nonhuman animals have "superior capacities, both actual and potential, for rationality, self-consciousness, communication, and anything else that can plausibly be considered morally significant" (1983, p.129). Human beings cannot be judged superior beings just because they are human beings. To take this viewpoint, Singer concluded, is to be a racist.

Are infants with severe disabilities unique? Singer argued that newborns cannot be regarded as distinct beings with lives of their own. Infants are not the same as persons. Because infants are somewhat inferior to people, killing them is not the same as killing a person.

Children with disabilities may have a life filled with pain and suffering and they may be unable to enjoy life as the typical person does. Many of these children are unwanted and they may be shifted from one foster home to another or from one residential facility to another. Many face years of medical care, perform poorly in school, and have difficulty locating meaningful work. Because of the difficulties of raising a child with severe disabilities, the family has a lower quality of life.

The quality of life of family members of infants who are disabled can be a concern because of the presumed physical, emotional, and economical stresses on the family. The demands of raising a child who is disabled may be difficult for certain families to manage. Some parents who consider the welfare of other individuals in the family and the pressures of having a child with a disability in the family may conclude that the sacrifices required of themselves and of other family members are not worth making when compared to the benefits of raising a child who is disabled (Duff & Campbell, 1973).

But the quality of life arguments demand that judgments are placed on degrees of quality. Which lives have more quality? Jonathan Glover (1977), using a hypothetical example, questioned the influence of judgments about the relative quality of the lives of persons when making treatment decisions:

> In one hospital a man given intensive care turned out to be a tramp and a meths drinker, and some people wondered if it would have been better to have provided the care for someone else. But even here it is hard to be sure how much the implied judgment of the quality of the man's life was influenced by mere social distance. I know very little about meths drinkers, and those who know more may have good reason for thinking their lives to be unhappy. But, if the doubts were partly based on the fact that the man was a tramp, we ought to be very suspicious of them (p.223).

Glover also pointed out that sorting people into categories of quality of life is a task that should be avoided:

> The less we sort people into different grades the better, especially given the fallibility of our judgments about the quality of people's lives. But again it seems doctrinaire to rule out the possibility of ever allowing weight to the sort of life the saved person can expect. If we accept that some people have lives so terrible as to be not worth living, it seems hard to deny the existence of a neighbouring grey area where a life may be worth living but is less worth living than normal. It would clearly be absurd to give priority in life-saving to someone whose life is not worth living. Yet it is hard, without making an artificially sharp cut-off point, to accept this while refusing to be influenced in selection by the fact that someone is in a state only a little less bad (1977, pp.223-224).

Has the quality of life improved for persons with severe disabilities? Powell and Hecimovic (1985) argued that the quality of life for persons with severe disabilities has advanced in the areas of education, social relationships, residential living, access, and technology. Early intervention programs as well as developments in rehabilitation and technology have enhanced the quality of life for persons with disabilities. These advances, although probably not widely understood or accepted, have greatly improved the lives of infants who are born disabled today, compared with children with disabilities who were born 10 years ago.

Federal and state legislation has also helped to improve the quality of life of persons with disabilities. On the federal level, the Architectural Barriers Act of 1968 is intended to make public buildings accessible. Section 504 of the Rehabilitation Act of 1973 requires that any program or activity that receives federal monies must be nondiscriminatory.

A free appropriate public education is guaranteed to all children with handicaps under The Education for All Handicapped Children Act, passed in 1975. The Developmental Disabilities Assistance and Bill of Rights Act, which was enacted in 1988, provides that all persons who have developmental disabilities may receive services to help them reach their potential.

C. Everett Koop (1989) acknowledged that medical predictions about the survival of children with disabilities have "seen a complete reversal of success and failure. When I first began in the field of pediatric surgery in 1946, most of the things that now have a 95 percent survival rate had a 95 percent mortality, and indeed, some carried a 100 percent mortality" (p.34).

In the case of Baby Jane Doe, inaccurate predictions about her progress were made shortly after her birth. Several physicians felt that she would never make much progress. Yet, at 4 years of age, this child was able to interact in a meaningful way with her parents and was attending school (U.S. Commission on Civil Rights, 1989).

PROVIDING TREATMENT

The principles of justice and equal treatment and certain beliefs about Christianity and God formed the basis of Paul Ramsey's (1978) arguments. He believed that only God knows how to be God and that as human beings we can never know the many reasons why God chooses to do things:

> But there is no indication at all that God is a rationalist whose care is a function of indicators of our personhood, or of our achievement within those capacities. He makes his rain to fall upon the just and the unjust alike, and his sun to rise on the abnormal as well as the normal. Indeed, he has special care for the weak and the vulnerable among us earth people. He cares according to need, not capacity or merit (Ramsey, 1978, p.205).

Ramsey opposed making distinctions between those infants who will live and those who will die based on criteria including consideration of the infant's medical diagnosis and outlook as well as socioeconomic and family variables. Neither an infant's family's poverty nor the parents' unstable marriage is reason for withholding vigorous treatment. According to Ramsey, "to deliberately make medical care a function of inequities that exist at birth is evidently to add injustice to injury and fate" (Ramsey, 1978, p.202).

Because of the principle of equality, concerns about personhood are irrelevant. The only medical criteria for providing care should be "physiological" (Ramsey, 1978, p.206). When treatment decisions are made, concerns about the normality or the abnormality of the infant should be rejected. Treatment should be provided regardless of the severity of the condition.

Dismissing considerations about the worthwhileness of an infant's life, Ramsey believed that it is impractical to compare the life of someone who is normal with the life of a person who has a severe disability. Rather, the comparison should be made between life and no life at all. But "no one can look into the chasm of life and death and weigh the difference" (Ramsey, 1978, p.207).

There are several possible exceptions to the position of providing treatment to all infants regardless of the severity of their medical conditions. Ramsey did not consider infants with anencephaly as being "born alive" (p.213) because these infants lack brain function. Although they are human, they are similar to patients who are brain dead. Thus, just as medical treatments are withheld from patients who are brain dead, treatment can be withheld from newborns with anencephaly. Although infants with anencephaly should not be considered alive, Ramsey believed that they should be given respect and that they should be allowed to "die all the way," rather than being assisted in dying (1978, p.214).

The second exception Ramsey (1978) made is for infants with Tay-Sachs disease. These infants endure a great deal of suffering while they are in the process of dying. For these infants, Ramsey suggested that the distinction between providing care and directly assisting these infants to die should be abolished.

Finally, because life for children who are born with Lesch-Nyhan syndrome is filled with agonized suffering and because there is no treatment, these infants can be assisted in dying:

> Is this not a close approximation to the insurmountable pain which in the terminal adult patient places him beyond human caring action and abolishes the more significance of the distinction between always continuing to care and direct dispatch? When care cannot be conveyed, it need not be extended (Ramsey, 1978, p.215).

Is there a distinction between abortion after the diagnosis of a birth defect and euthanasia of a newborn with a severe handicap? According to John C. Fletcher (1974; 1975; 1979; 1982), these can be considered separately because of differences in development and in circumstances.

Fletcher maintained that there are three critical differences: a) unlike the fetus, an infant is biologically separate from the mother; b) it is easier to treat an infant who is critically ill than a fetus; and, c) parents more readily accept an infant as a "real person" (1975, p.76) than a fetus.

In addition, Fletcher believed that the practice of euthanasia brutalizes those who participate in it. He also maintained that to permit euthanasia to be practiced is to change "the ethical ambience of the birth of infants from one of thorough caring for life to one in which the public accepted a policy of euthanasia and supported its legalization" (Fletcher, 1975, p.77). Based on these arguments, Fletcher opposed euthanasia of infants who are critically ill.

The only circumstances under which pediatric euthanasia would be acceptable are described in a hypothetical situation. Several people live on a remote island where there is little food and the living conditions are severe. There are at least two expectant mothers and one of the mothers has given birth to a child who has a severe disability. If there is little food and other children might starve, euthanasia of the newborn would be permitted in order to allow the older children to survive.

John C. Fletcher (1982) maintained that physicians are not taught about euthanasia and that killing a child would cause additional suffering and guilt in the parents. He wrote that the strongest argument against killing is that it "is a denial of the help that God gives" (1982, p.96).

> Human survival is rooted more in the long run in trust in a Creator of life than on the ethical powers of humans to reason about the conditions under which survival can be justified. The 'courage to be' does not finally arise from debatable ethical beliefs, but from trust in an indestructible source of mercy (agape) that is incompatible with a practice of killing human beings who are suffering (Fletcher, 1982, p.96).

There are theological reasons for the birth of a child with a genetic disorder. God not only is creative and redemptive but also emancipative. God is "mighty and good" (Fletcher, 1982, p.171) and saves us from the awful fate of not making any difference at all. God intends that there be a greater amount of good than evil in the world and "God intends that all creatures be emancipated from any form of bondage that threatens to subvert the creative limits of natural order" (p.171). Humans need to participate in this work of emancipation and salvation.

Boyle (1982) rejected any considerations about the quality of life as a rationale for active or passive euthanasia. He believed that using quality of life standards violates the inherent rights of patients. The right to life is just as valid for incompetent patients and seriously ill newborns as it is for any other patient. It is discriminatory to hold one set of standards for a competent person and another set of standards for an incompetent person or a seriously ill infant.

The thrust of Boyle's argument is that when making life and death decisions about seriously ill newborns, the issue of fairness must be of prime importance. In order to ensure fairness, the parents and family of the infants, along with the physician must make the treatment decisions.

Although Shelp (1986) believed that parents should also make treatment decisions for their children, he argued that parents, philosophically, historically, legally, and theologically, have the authority to make decisions not to treat their children when one of the following conditions exist:

> (1) extended life is reasonably judged not to constitute a net benefit to the infant; (2) it is reasonably believed that the infant's condition is such that the capacities sufficient for a minimal independent existence or personhood in a strict sense cannot be attained; or (3) the costs to other persons, especially parents and family, are sufficient to defeat customary duties of beneficence toward a particular human infant (Shelp, 1986, p.203).

Shelp maintained that newborns are persons in a "social sense" rather than a "strict sense." In making this distinction, he wrote that newborns:

> do not possess the properties or capacities sufficient for unqualified membership in the moral community, are not morally self-determining, or bearers of rights and duties, including those of forbearance and beneficence (1986, p.203).

Newborns are persons in a social sense because of their place in the moral order. Parents hold the rights and duties of their children for them until they are ready to take these rights and duties upon themselves. Because of the moral order, parents have the authority to care for and to make decisions for their offspring.

What consideration should be given to parental rights? Garland (1977) conceptualized the types of decisions that parents make when their newborn is critically ill. He reasoned that, although all infants have an equal right to life, this right does not outweigh parental rights or the needs of the family that must be considered when making treatment decisions about seriously ill newborns.

There are three types of decisions that can be made when parents have a critically ill newborn: the infant must receive treatment; the infant may be treated or may be allowed to die, depending on the decision of the parents; and the infant should be allowed to die. Garland believes that parents must be involved in all three of these types of decisions. In the first decision, parental permission is regarded as a formality because the infant has the right to life. For the second decision, parents must consider the needs of the family and avoid putting the family under any insurmountable hardships. For the third decision, parents have a duty to withhold treatment. Here, the parents should consider the best interests of the newborn and their obligation not to do harm. By prolonging the life of their critically ill child, they may be doing harm to the infant.

A somewhat different means of arriving at a medical decision, one that is based on a series of moral principles, has been proposed by Coburn (1980). He suggested that the way to resolve treatment dilemmas is to construct a hypothetical situation in which a moral legislator chooses a plan of action without knowing anything about the infant or the circumstances surrounding its birth. This is the only way to make sure that the medical decision that is made is impartial and unbiased.

There are four moral principles that an impartial legislator would choose to use when making medical treatment decisions. These principles rest on three tenets: whether the life of the newborn will be worth living; the net benefits of the death of the infant; and the amount of suffering the newborn will endure prior to reaching "the age of reason" (Coburn, 1980, p.354). Two of these principles state the conditions under which it is not permitted to end the life of the newborn:

1. It is impermissible to terminate the life of a defective newborn, actively or passively, when it is the case that (a) it cannot be concluded beyond any reasonable doubt that the infant would be better off dead, even if (b) it will be replaced by a child whose life prospects are better—even significantly better—and (c) its death will confer significant net benefits on those most directly affected by it.

2. It is also impermissible to terminate the life of a defective newborn, either actively or passively, when (a) there is good reason for thinking that its life will not be worth living, even if (b) its death will confer significant net benefits on those most directly affected by it, provided (c) it will not undergo significant amounts of suffering prior to reaching 'the age of reason' (Coburn, 1980, p.354).

The third and fourth principles outline the moral principles which are permissible when making treatment decisions:

3. It is, however, permissible to terminate the life of a defective newborn, either actively or passively, when there is good reason for thinking (a) that it will not survive the first several years of life, (b) that during those years its experiences will either be of no value to it or mainly negative, and (c) its death will confer significant net benefits on those most directly affected by it.

4. It is also permissible to terminate the life of a defective newborn, either actively or passively, when there is good reason for thinking (a) its life will not be worth living, (b) it will undergo significant amounts of suffering prior to reaching 'the age of reason,' and (c) its death will confer significant net benefits on those most directly affected by it (Coburn, 1980, p.354).

BEST INTERESTS

The principle of beneficence holds that physicians do no harm and provide treatment whenever possible. Is it beneficial to prolong the lives of infants who, although remaining alive, will experience and feel little? It can be argued that neither Karen Ann Quinlan, who remained in a coma for almost 10 years, nor her family benefitted from having her life lengthened. Karen Ann Quinlan was not aware that her life was prolonged and the suffering of her family was exacerbated. Is it beneficial to impose on the parents of fetuses and infants with severe disabilities a lifetime of care and financial commitment?

In an historic article, Duff and Campbell (1973) openly acknowledged that decisions not to treat infants with severe disabilities occur frequently in neonatal intensive care units. While their position has evolved over the years, Duff and Campbell (1987), wrote that they advocate a "family-centered policy" when making treatment decisions for critically ill newborns. Relying on their experiences of caring for critically ill newborns in intensive care units, they believed that treatment decisions should be made by "moral communities" comprised of intimate members of each persons family and their advisors in concert with health care providers. These moral communities should make decisions: whether or not to use technology; the extent to which technology should be used; when and how resuscitation should be attempted; and how care should be given to a person who has a poor prognosis. In addition, they argued that the results of medical and care interventions should be reviewed by health professionals:

> In the overall scheme of care, health professionals should try to persuade their clients to accept treatment when prognosis with treatment is improved and life seems really promising. That is an easy task. They should try to persuade their clients to forego treatment (but yet continue caring) when treatment is futile and prognosis hopeless. That is a more difficult task, often requiring the passage of time. When prognosis is such that the benefits of treatment are much in doubt and treatment may cause more harm than non-treatment, clients should be invited to wrestle with these ambiguities and decide with professional advisors what choices best fulfill their duties to the sick and their loyalties to principles of justice, utility, and possibly other values (Duff & Campbell, 1987, p.284).

Mahowald (1986) wrote that there are three principles or values that must be considered when making ethical decisions about newborns: beneficence, autonomy, and justice. The principle that should have top priority is beneficence. Beneficence toward the infant should be considered before beneficence toward others. But kindness toward the infant does not mean that the interests of others are dismissed. Respect must be given for the autonomy of all of the persons who are involved in the ethical decision. The principle of justice must be applied when considering these interests. Mahowald maintained that the persons involved with ethical decisions should be included in the following order: parents, physicians, health care team members, hospital ethics committees, and the courts.

About beneficence, Mahowald wrote:

With regard to each infant, beneficence entails concern for both immediate and long-range needs; these are often inseparable from consideration of the family and social supports upon which the child depends. In certain tragic circumstances, this principle entails recognition of the fact that caring extends beyond curing, and affirmation of the right to die as part of an individual's right to live (Mahowald, 1986, p.82).

THE CHILD ABUSE
AMENDMENTS OF 1984

The Child Abuse Amendments of 1984 provide that states that receive federal financial assistance for child abuse and neglect programs must provide protection to infants with disabilities. The Child Abuse Amendments mandate that all infants with disabilities receive nutrition, hydration, and medication and that all infants with disabilities must be given medically indicated treatment, with three exceptions:

1. The infant is chronically and irreversibly comatose;
2. The provision of such treatment would merely prolong dying, not be effective in ameliorating or correcting all of the infant's life-threatening conditions, or otherwise be futile in terms of the survival of the infant;
3. The provision of such treatment would be virtually futile in terms of the survival of the infant and the treatment itself under such circumstances would be inhumane (Federal Register, 1985, p.479).

A high standard of care must be provided to infants with disabilities and the treatment must be likely to be effective. However, numerous violations of the Child Abuse Amendments of 1984 have been documented (U.S. Commission on Civil Rights, 1989). The U.S. Commission on Civil Rights concluded that, "If adequately enforced, the law would provide strong protection for many children with disabilities against denial of lifesaving treatment" (1989, p.7).

IMPACT ON SOCIETY

Medical care for critically ill infants is extremely expensive. The Office of Technology Assessment (U.S. Congress, 1987) estimated that the average cost in a neonatal intensive care unit for a low birthweight baby is between $31,000 and $71,000. Many of the babies whose mothers abused drugs or alcohol are born prematurely, and their mothers had little or no prenatal care. Some are born with AIDS or other chronic debilitating illnesses.

The tiniest babies stay in the hospital the longest. For these babies, the average costs are between $62,000 and $150,000. For some infants, the costs can be more than $500,000 (Gustaitis & Young, 1986; Lyon, 1985). More than

$2 billion was spent in 1985 for neonatal intensive care for 200,000 critically ill babies. These 200,000 infants represented about six percent of all babies born in that year (Gustaitis & Young, 1986).

Some of the infants who started out under fragile circumstances have or will develop disabilities. Many infants will require a great deal of medical and supportive care when they are young. As they grow older, many more community and school resources will have to be mobilized to educate, care for, and support them.

As adults, some may be able to hold jobs, others may require supportive employment, and still others may require almost total care. It has been estimated that it will cost $15 billion dollars to prepare drug-addicted babies for kindergarten and $6 billion dollars to educate them through high school (Labaton, 1989). The federal budget for the education of children with disabilities for 1990 was $2,055,255,000.

Intensive care medicine can be very lucrative for hospitals (Gustaitis & Young, 1986). In addition to the money generated for each crib in an intensive care unit, hospitals earn a great deal of money from laboratory tests, CAT scans, and other high technology procedures. Thus, aside from humanitarian efforts, the drive to expand neonatal intensive care, according to Gustaitis and Young (1986), is fueled by the economic benefits to a hospital. While some cost-benefit analyses show that, from an economic perspective, it is unsound to fund neonatal intensive care, especially for babies who weigh less than 750 grams, hospitals continue to expand their neonatal intensive care units.

Many babies are abandoned in hospitals. Some children must live in hospitals because there is no place for them to go, or they may move from one foster home or residential facility to another. These are the children who remain unadopted. Society is left with the responsibility of providing nurture, shelter, food, education, and medical care.

The trend toward caring for persons with disabilities in group homes rather than in large residential centers has helped to mediate some of the staggering costs. Financial incentives, which will also assist in reducing costs, would aid families and persons with disabilities to be cared for in their own homes. The development of community-based employment opportunities and supported employment will help to raise the productivity levels of persons with disabilities. The isolation and segregation of persons with disabilities makes it much more expensive and difficult to include them in the mainstream of economic life (U.S. Commission on Civil Rights, 1989).

Kuhse, MacKenzie, and Singer (1988) believed that too much money is being spent on neonatal intensive care. They proposed that much of the money that is budgeted for neonatal intensive care should be reallocated to providing prenatal care to women who are at risk of giving birth to premature or low birthweight babies. They propose somewhat of a triage policy, with certain infants being allowed into intensive care, and others being denied intensive care. Babies would be divided into five groups:

1. Automatically eligible for NICU (neonatal intensive care unit) treatment.
2. Eligible on written recommendation of attending physician, giving reasons.
3. Referred to NICU eligibility committee.
4. May be excluded from NICU on written recommendation of attending physician, giving reasons.
5. Ineligible for NICU treatment. Babies with intraventricular hemorrhage with intracranial extension, or babies born weighing less than 750 g who require mechanical ventilation from birth, may simply be ineligible (class 5). Babies born weighing more than 1500 g who do not suffer from any of a short list of conditions may be automatically eligible if their parents give informed consent, as for any other medical treatment (class 1). Between these two classes may be criteria which indicate eligibility (and ineligibility) conditional upon the attending clinician's consulting with the child's parents and submitting, to an ethics committee or similar body, a short statement of reasons for the decisions. Between those classes too, there would be intermediates. (Kuhse et.al., 1988, p.238).

Many studies have attempted to define and quantify quality of life (Emery & Schneiderman, 1989; Mukerjee, 1989). Mukerjee (1989) wrote that research into the quality of life has spread all over the world. Some theorists have developed the concept of a QALY, which is a year of healthy life expectancy (Williams, 1985). Various mathematical formulas have been developed that are intended to aid in making medical care decisions about quality of life and life expectancy. Williams (1985) wrote that positive amounts of QALYs are produced by beneficial health care activities. Health care activities that have high priority have a low cost for each QALY; health care activities that have a lower importance have a higher cost for each QALY. Various illnesses and disabilities are rated and the value of a QALY can be computed for them.

The dilemma of how to quantify or ascribe a value to quality of life was also addressed by Shaw (1988). He developed an equation to aid in making decisions about critically ill persons of any age. The equation states:

QL = NE × (H+S) where: QL = Quality of Life; NE = Natural Endowment; H = Contributions by Home (Family); S = Contributions by Society.

Recognizing that this equation can be used as a means of justifying nontreatment of infants with severe disabilities or of rationalizing the withholding of resources, Shaw believed that this formula is helpful because it can be used within the context of each unique situation in order to better understand the decision making process. He believed that this equation should not be computed, but should be used to assist in making decisions.

Shaw wrote that this formula has been criticized as a "prescription for infanticide" (1988, p.11) and as a means "to justify nontreatment of impaired infants on the basis of a predicted low QL, which is itself the predictable consequence of withholding resources by family and/or society" (p.11).

But he maintained that the formula does not provide information on whether treatment should be provided, withdrawn, or withheld. The formula should be considered within the context of each situation. It is not above moral discussions about the quality of life; it only helps in the understanding of the decision making process.

The application of quality of life criteria has been condemned by the U.S. Commission on Civil Rights:

> The bases typically advanced to support denial of lifesaving medical treat-
> ment, food, and fluids based on disability—that the quality of life of a person
> with a disability will be unacceptably poor, or that such a person's continued
> existence will impose an unacceptable burden on his family or the Nation,
> as a whole—are often grounded in misinformation, inaccurate stereotypes,
> and negative attitudes about people with disabilities (1989, p.47).

Cost-effectiveness analysis is a recent approach that is also supposed to assist in making medical care decisions. All cost-effectiveness formulas have similar components (Emery & Schneiderman, 1989, p.8):

$$\frac{\text{Monetary Cost (D)}-\text{Monetary Benefits (D)}}{\text{Health Gained (D)}}$$
$$D = \text{discounting of future values.}$$

In this approach, monetary costs include funds for all medical treatments, such as diagnosis, medical care, and rehabilitation. The costs of any side effects are also calculated, as well as any long-term costs. The benefits are generally calculated as wages earned. The health gained is measured by a shorter hospital stay, decrease in the death rate, and the lengthening or shortening of the life span.

Cost-effectiveness analysis when employed by policy makers can be used to determine the effectiveness of certain intervention programs. These include: comparing different treatments; deciding the best use of funds that have been targeted for specific populations; determining which under-funded treatments or programs should be funded; and identifying medical programs that are not cost effective (Emery & Schneiderman, 1989).

Strong (1983) wrote that the costs of caring for very low birthweight babies are not unreasonable. When compared with other federal expenditures, the costs associated with the care of these babies is small. She wrote:

> This relatively small part of the tax bill seems not too high a price to pay in
> order to avoid the apparent injustice that would be involved in not trying
> to save these infants. Furthermore, with regard to individual cases, whatever
> limit there may be to a right to health care would presumably not be reached
> in the early days of treatment (1983, p.18).

In a pessimistic examination of health care costs in the United States, Callahan (1988) asserted that some patients will not receive the same quality of care as other patients. He wrote that a realistic view of escalating health care costs means that different patients will receive differential treatments and that rationing of health care must be considered. The emphasis on individual rights must give way to the well-being of the community, and this will mean that individuals will have to sacrifice health care. "The present system of focusing on individual needs leaves no room for the broader needs of the community as a whole, no room for anything less than crude trade-off thinking in moments of pressure and no room for placing health needs within some broader perspective of the full scope of many other human needs" (Callahan, 1988, p.20).

The U.S. Commission on Civil Rights (1989) wrote that the real costs of disabilities are in the policies that promote the segregation and isolation of persons with disabilities:

> The assumption has been that the level of severity of disability is the major determinant of lifetime costs and, consequently, that the more severely disabled a child may appear to be at birth, the less likely it is that the child will be able to contribute as an adult to his or her own economic sufficiency and the more expensive it will be to meet that person's basic needs. Although this assumption is unfounded, it has resulted in a self-fulfilling prophecy: a diagnosis of severe disability leads to placement of a person in an institutional and nonwork environment that significantly limits that person's capability and entails far more expense than necessary (p.55).

DIFFICULT DECISIONS

What should be the best course of action for critically ill babies? Is it preferable to take the sanctity of life view and provide treatment at all costs without regard for the outcome? Should the quality of life of the infant and of the family be considerations? What course of action is in the best interests of the child and the family? What value should be placed on the possibility that this child has a disability? What weight should be given to the impact of the staggering costs of caring for these children on society? These and other complex questions remain before us.

In the United States, physicians are trained to provide aggressive treatment. For some infants who are hopelessly ill, the process of dying will be extended. The family may endure months of emotional agony and may see their financial resources drained. Numerous social, educational, and financial resources may have to be mobilized throughout the life of the survivors.

One of the difficulties of considering each of the ethical viewpoints in arriving at decisions is that each uses different vocabulary, assumptions, and conceptualizations. How can common standards or criteria be developed? Many of the writers use abstractions. What happens when an actual child is involved? Can abstract philosophical arguments be applied to real life situations? Overlaying the difficulties of arriving at a common understanding of the positions is the political arena. Cost-effectiveness analysis and quality of life formulas can be biased against seriously ill newborns. Quantitative analysis, when used as a justification to deny treatment, is discriminatory (U.S. Commission on Civil Rights, 1989). The costs of caring for an infant should never be considered when making treatment decisions.

Because the outcomes for many of these infants are unclear, an estimate of the potential wages that might be earned is difficult to calculate. In addition, the costs of intensive care are high at the beginning of life and may continue for an extended period of time. Society may never be able to reap the benefits, in real dollars, of keeping these infants alive.

When the costs of neonatal intensive care are compared with the costs of other programs, such as prenatal care, treatment for patients with AIDS, and long-term care of the elderly, it becomes increasingly difficult to make choices. Inequalities exist in the distribution of resources. The challenge in a democratic society is to provide justice and equality for all. Is this possible?

These are hard decisions. Which approach provides the best course of action? The debates will continue but Rhoden (1986) emphasized that these ethical dilemmas must be faced:

> There will be ghosts, and there will be profoundly retarded, crib-bound survivors, but our society will have even more explaining to do if we blind ourselves to the tragic and complex nature of these choices in the newborn nursery (Rhoden, 1986, p.42).

REFERENCES

Angell, M. (1988). Euthanasia. *The New England Journal of Medicine, 319,* 1348-1350.

Boyle, J. M. (1982). Treating defective newborns: Who decides? On what basis? *Hospital Progress, 636,* 34-37, 61.

Bridge, P., & Bridge, M. (1981). The brief life and death of Christopher Bridge. *The Hastings Center Report, 11,* 17-19.

Callahan, D. (1988). Allocating health resources. *The Hastings Center Report, 18,* 14-20.

Child Abuse Amendments of 1984. P.L. 98-457 (98 Stat.) 1749-1757.

Coburn, R.C. (1980). Morality and the defective newborn. *The Journal of Medicine and Philosophy, 5,* 340-357.

Devlin, D., & Magrab, P.R. (1981). Bioethical considerations in the care of handicapped newborns. *Journal of Pediatric Psychology, 6,* 111-119.

Duff, R. (1978). Deciding the care of defective infants. In M. Kohl (Ed.), *Infanticide and the value of life* (pp.96-101). Buffalo: Prometheus Books.

Duff, R., & Campbell, G. (1973). Moral and ethical dilemmas in the special care nursery. *The New England Journal of Medicine, 289,* 890-894.

Duff, R., & Campbell, G. (1976). On deciding the care of severely handicapped or dying persons: With particular reference to infants. *Pediatrics, 57,* 487-493.

Duff, R., & Campbell, G. (1987). Moral communities and tragic choices. In R. C. Mcmillan, H. T. Engelhardt, Jr., & S. F. Spicker (Eds.), *Euthanasia and the newborn* (pp.273-289). Dordrecht, Holland: D. Reidel.

Emery, D. D., & Schneiderman, L. J. (1989). Cost-effectiveness analysis in health care. *The Hastings Center Report*, *19*, 8-13.

English, J. (1975). Abortion and the concept of a person. In N. Quist (Ed.), *The rights of the fetus* (pp.418-431). Frederick, MD: University Publications of America.

Federal Register (1985, April 15). Child abuse and neglect prevention and treatment program; Final rule. Vol. 50, No. 72, 469-492.

Fletcher, J. (1978). Infanticide and the ethics of loving concern. In M. Kohl (Ed.), *Infanticide and the value of life* (pp.13-22). Buffalo: Prometheus Books.

Fletcher, J.C. (1974). Attitudes toward defective newborns. *The Hastings Center Studies*, *2*, 21-32.

Fletcher, J.C. (1975). Abortion, euthanasia, and care of defective newborns. *New England Journal of Medicine*, *292*, 75-78.

Fletcher, J.C. (1979). Prenatal diagnosis, selective abortion and the ethics of withholding treatment from the defective newborn. In A. Capron, M. Loppe, R.F. Murray, T. Powledge, S. Twiss, & D. Bergsma (Eds.), *Abortion: Moral and Legal Perspectives*. Amherst: The University of Massachusetts Press.

Fletcher, J.C. (1982). *Coping with genetic disorders*. San Francisco: Harper & Row.

Garland, M. J. (1977). Care of the newborn: the decision not to treat. *Perinatology/Neonatolgy*, *15*, 14-21, 43-44.

Glover, J. (1977). *Causing death and saving lives*. Reading, England: Penguin.

Gustafson, J.M. (1973). Mongolism, parental desires, and the right to life. *Perspectives in Biology and Medicine*, *16*, 529-557.

Gustaitis, R., & Young, E. W. D. (1986). *A Time to Be Born, A Time to Die*. Reading, MA: Addison Wesley.

Jakobovits, I. (1978). Jewish views on infanticide. In M. Kohl (Ed.), *Infanticide and the value of life* (pp.23-31). Buffalo: Prometheus Books.

Kevles, D. J. (1985). *In the Name of Eugenics*. New York: Alfred A. Knopf.

Kluge, E. (1980). The euthanasia of radically defective neonates: Some statutory considerations. *Dalhousie Law Review*, *6*, 229-257.

Koop, C. E. (1985). Protection of Handicapped Newborns: Hearing Before the United States Commission on Civil Rights 7-8. Testimony of Surgeon General, U.S. Public Health Service. (Cited by the U.S. Commission on Civil Rights, 1989. *Medical discrimination against children with disabilities*. Washington, DC: U.S. Commission on Civil Rights, p.34.)

Kuhse, H., MacKenzie, J., & Singer, P. (1988). Allocating resources in perinatal medicine: A proposal. *Australian Pediatric Journal*, *24*, 235-239.

Labaton, S. (1989, December 5). The cost of drug abuse: $60 billion a year. *The New York Times*, pp.D1, D6.

Lyon, J. (1985). *Playing God in the nursery*. New York: W. W. Norton Co.

Mahowald, M.B. (1986). Ethical decisions in neonatal intensive care. In S. J. Youngner (Ed.), *Human values in critical care medicine* (pp.63-86). New York: Praeger.

McCormick, M. C. (1985). The contribution of low birth weight to infant mortality and childhood morbidity. *Journal of the American Medical Association*, *261*, 1761-1772.

Mukherjee, R. (1989). *The Quality of Life*. New Delhi, India: Sage.

Powell, T., & Hecimovic, A. (1985). Baby Doe and the search for quality of life. *Exceptional Children*, *51* (4), 315-523.

Rachels, J. (1975). Active and passive euthanasia. *The New England Journal of Medicine*, *292*, 78-80.

Ramsey, P. (1978). Ethics at the edges of life. New Haven: Yale University Press.

Rhoden, N. K. (1986). Treating baby Doe: The ethics of uncertainty. *The Hastings Center Report*, *16*, 34-42.

Robertson, J. A. (1975). Involuntary euthanasia of defective newborns: A legal analysis. *Stanford Law Review*, *27*, 213-269.

Shaw, A. (1988). QL revisited. *The Hastings Center Report*, *18*, 10-12.

Shelp, E. E. (1986). *Born to die? Deciding the fate of critically ill newborns*. New York: Free Press.

Singer, P. (1979). *Practical ethics*. Cambridge, England: Cambridge University Press.

Singer, P. (1983). Sanctity of life or quality of life. *Pediatrics*, *72*, 128-129.

Strong, C. (1983). The tiniest newborns. *The Hastings Center Report*, *13*, 14-19.

Taub, S. J. D. (1982). Withholding treatment from defective newborns. *American Society of Law and Medicine*, *10*, 4-10.

Tooley, M. (1979). Decision to terminate life and the concept of person. In J. Ladd (Ed.), *Ethical issues relating to life and death,* (pp.62-93). New York: Oxford University Press.

Tooley, M. (1983). *Abortion and infanticide.* Oxford: Clarendon Press.

U.S. Commission on Civil Rights (1989). *Medical discrimination aginst children with disabilities.* Washington, D C: U.S. Commission on Civil Rights.

U.S. Congress, Office of Technology Assessment (1987). *Neonatal intensive care for low birthweight infants: Costs and effectiveness* (Health Technology Case Study 38). Washington, DC: U.S. Congress, Office of Technology Assessment.

Williams, A. (1985). The value of QALYs. *Health and Social Service Journal, 95,* (4957), unpaged.

Chapter 6

Neonatal Intensive Care

Upon entering an intensive care unit, the visitor is startled. Bright lights shine day and night; there is a din caused by the monitors and high technology machines. Incubators, intravenous tubes, and monitoring equipment abound. Nurses watch the machines and provide care; physicians check the charts and the patients. At the center of all of this technology are the tiniest, most fragile newborns who are struggling to survive. The babies, some of whom look no different from a fetus, lay in isolettes, bassinets, cribs, or on slanted hotbeds warmed by radiant lamps. The smallest babies have arms that are not any bigger than their mother's finger; their heels are as tiny as a pencil eraser. The blood volume of each baby is approximately six tablespoons (Gustaitis & Young, 1986).

In the U.S., the delivery of intensive care medicine can be characterized as aggressive and vigorous. When a life is in the balance, the typical response is to begin life-saving treatment immediately and to use all the technology that is available. Neonatal care medicine is no exception. This chapter will examine the consequences of the delivery of high technology medicine in neonatal intensive care units on the babies, the care givers, and the families.

THE BABIES

As of 1983, there were approximately 534 hospitals in the United States that had neonatal intensive care units, with a total of 7,684 beds (U. S. Congress, 1987). Approximately 200,000 newborns are admitted to these units each year, with an estimated length of stay between 8 and 18 days for each.

The hospitals that have neonatal intensive units form a loosely connected system and are categorized into three levels of intensive care. The hospitals in Level I provide normal newborn care; Level II hospitals provide intensive care but do not have the full range of services of Level III hospitals; and Level III hospitals are usually regional centers that provide the most intensive care (U. S. Congress, 1987; Weir, 1984).

Inadequate prenatal care, poor nutrition (Strong, 1983), and the use of drugs by the mother all contribute to premature birth and poor fetal growth. Infants who are born after the 27th or 28th week of pregnancy stand a good chance of survival; many of the infants who are born before the 25th week of pregnancy do not live. Infants who are born before the 24th week of pregnancy have lungs that are too immature to permit them to survive (Gustaitis & Young, 1986).

About 75,000 to 100,000 low birthweight babies are admitted to neonatal intensive care units each year. This number represents approximately one half of all of the admissions to neonatal intensive care units (U.S. Congress, 1987).

Although gestational age is more likely to influence the well-being of the infant, birthweight is a more reliable measure. Infants who weigh less than 2,500 grams at birth are called low birthweight babies. Very low birthweight infants weigh less than 1,500 grams at birth, and these account for approximately 1.15% of all babies born. Extremely low birthweight babies weigh less than 1,000 grams at birth. (McCormick, 1985; U. S. Congress, 1987).

Recent attention has focused on infants who weigh less than 1,000 grams at birth. Many of these babies suffer from major medical problems, including hyaline membrane disease, a lung disease caused by immature lungs; asphyxia, lack of oxygen that can cause brain damage and lead to brain hemorrhage; hypothermia; hypoglycemia; infections; jaundice; congenital problems; and cardiac disease (McCormick, 1985; Strong, 1983).

Besides being at increased risk of mortality and morbidity, low birthweight babies are in danger of developing long-term disability. The Office of Technology Assessment (U.S. Congress, 1987) has estimated that of the infants who are admitted to neonatal intensive care units, 27% will die, 16% will be seriously or moderately disabled, and 57% will develop normally. In addition, low birthweight babies may be at increased risk of child abuse.

With vigorous medical treatment, the majority of critically ill babies survive. For many of these babies, the treatment that keeps them alive can also injure them. In addition, there is some concern that the physical environment of the intensive care unit, with its strong lighting and high noise levels, can be detrimental to the well-being of these babies. Just taking several blood samples each day can deplete an infant's small blood supply.

Aside from a long hospitalization at birth, many of these babies are rehospitalized during infancy. Along with the hospitalizations are increased visits by the physician, increased medical services, higher medical costs, and a major impact on the functioning of the family (McCormick, 1985).

There is still much that we do not know about the survivors of neonatal intensive care units. Additional research on morbidity, mortality, and outcomes is needed. While the effectiveness of neonatal intensive care units is apparent, the longitudinal benefits of certain types of interventions on specific children must be examined (McCormick, 1989).

Some of these infants will die; others will develop learning difficulties by the time they enter school (Klein, Hack, Gallagher, & Fanaroff, 1985; McCormick, 1985). In a study of 80 low birthweight infants who were evaluated when they were 5 years old, Klein et al., (1985) found that 15 children had IQs below 85 or had neurological impairments. Of the remaining children, those who were born with very low birthweights performed significantly poorer on tests of spatial and visual motor performance.

With respect to infants who survive with a disability, McCormick (1989) wrote that although most of the babies do not have a mild or moderate disability, the information about outcomes is scarce and:

> the need for special education services may also be increased in VLBW (very low birthweight) survivors in the school-aged period. The effect of these burdens on the families of school-aged children who were VLBW requires further examination (p.1771).

THE NURSES

The nurses who care for the tiny, fragile infants in the neonatal intensive care unit face enormous pressures. They work with high technology equipment, must react quickly, and care for infants who are on the edge of life. These nurses have to keep up a hectic pace; they must respond to crises quickly and efficiently. Working in an isolated environment that separates them from other nurses, they must operate complex equipment, and help families deal with their children, and they are chronically anxious because of the life-and-death nature of their work. Adding to the tension and the stress is the repetitive nature of their jobs and the fact that they face death daily (Lipsky, 1984).

Two groups, the physicians and the nurses, run the neonatal intensive care units. The job of the nurses is critical in three ways: they are responsible for the day-to-day routine of the neonatal intensive care unit; their work is emotionally and psychologically draining; and they frequently communicate with the parents (Weir, 1984). A nurse's daily routine in the neonatal intensive care unit can include the following:

> Nurses are responsible for evaluating the gestational age of new arrivals, stabilizing body temperature, watching for shock, carefully noting respiration and circulation, starting intravenous infusions, suctioning at a moment's notice (especially with infants receiving ventilatory assistance or premature infants whose secretions and vomit place them in danger of asphyxia), bathing the infants, feeding them, weighing them, providing oxygen for some of them, controlling infection (e.g., by thorough hand washing before and after handling an infant, wearing a cover gown whenever holding an infant), cleaning and disinfecting the neonate's living environment, and in every possible way immediately being aware of any significant change in a neonate's condition (House & Dombkiewicz, 1981, cited by Weir, 1984, pp.32-33).

In addition to the demanding physical care that nurses provide for these infants, there are ethical pressures:

> Substantive ethical issues in these instances include passive euthanasia, the 'rightness' of medical research, financial stress for the parents of the infant, complete informed consent, maximum uses of scarce or limited resources,

patient and parent advocacy, collegial relationship with physicians (Weise, 1981, p.53).

The care of these infants takes a great emotional toll on the nurses. For example, the nurses who cared for one infant who was born with an incurable illness were especially frustrated. They expressed "desperation" at having to care for an infant who "cries and screams" and was described as "unsocialized," "unrewarding," possibly "autistic," or "damaged" (Anspach, 1989, p.64). One of the nurses reflected:

> I think they should have stopped on her a long, long time before they did...and you can tell me, and they come along and say 'this little life can amount to something.' That doesn't...make the decision right, because sure, you don't know exactly what's going to happen, but you have a pretty good idea she's going to be damaged... She was psychologically damaged by the time she died. No one loved Robin for eight months of life. She was handled only when something had to be done to her. And it was her stiffness. Every time you would approach, she would become stiff and withdraw. She could feel the frustration in your hands. Finally, I just said, 'Well, I'll just gavage (feed by a tube to the stomach) you and leave you there in a corner' (Anspach, 1989, p.65).

Another case illustrates the emotional impact of caring for critically ill newborns on the nurses. One researcher, Fred M. Frohock (1986), spent four months as a participant observer in an intensive care nursery. He described his observations and interviews in his book, *Special Care*. One infant, Stephanie, particularly interested him. Despite Stephanie's prematurity, her medical problem was that she had a congenital disorder, epidermolysis bullosa, that caused constant blistering of the skin. While there was no scarring, the blistering was found on the outside of the body and on skin inside the body, such as the mouth and esophagus.

One of the nurses, interviewed after Stephanie died, was asked about the most difficult part in caring for Stephanie. In response, she voiced frustration and replied that it was very difficult to see Stephanie endure so much pain and be able to do so little to help to relieve it.

THE PHYSICIANS

Physicians are sometimes viewed as less emotionally involved than the nurses. They see their patients once or twice a day and, for the most part, do not participate in the physical care of the infants. While they may order certain procedures, it is the nurses who suction, change the dressings, and feed the infants. But they face other pressures. They must decide what types of interventions must be undertaken and whether ordinary or extraordinary means should be pursued.

The primary physician for Stephanie, when asked about deciding the course of treatment for her, expressed agony and frustration in making treatment decisions for a critically ill infant who had a condition for which there was no treatment and no cure.

Physicians must assess the infants, diagnose their medical problems, prescribe treatment, communicate the condition of the newborns to the parents, and consult with them and with other medical personnel about treatment. They may be involved in team meetings with nurses, community and religious leaders, and ethicists. They must be aware of the legal and ethical ramifications of their decisions.

The U.S. Commission on Civil Rights (1989) found that medical discrimination against infants with disabilities was prevalent and that doctors often encourage the denial of treatment. Doctors are frequently viewed as all powerful and all knowing by parents. The conveying of inaccurate information about the prognosis of an infant with a disability and the quality of life for persons with disabilities can influence treatment decisions that are made by the parents because they usually defer to the physician's decision.

THE PARENTS

The birth of a child with a disability or potential disability is very stressful for the parents. They may be angry, depressed, grief stricken, and guilty. Many of the them are provided inadequate information about the disability and the quality of life of a person with a disability. Because the parents may believe that their child will be a burden on the family, they may decide to deny treatment (U.S. Commission on Civil Rights, 1989).

A low birthweight infant can have a significant impact on the family. The attachment between the mother and the child can be affected; parents may become overprotective, physically abusive, and anxious. In addition, a low birthweight baby can affect marital stability, parental employment, the social contacts of the parents, vacations, and the behavior of other children in the family (McCormick, 1985).

The parents have little control over their child's referral to the neonatal intensive care unit and subsequent treatment. Once the child is a patient in the neonatal intensive care unit, the hospital staff may assume that the guardianship has passed to the physician. The staff has certain expectations for the behavior of the parents and one of them is to be grateful for caring for their infant (Guillemin & Holmstrom, 1986).

Although the staff of a neonatal intensive care unit is accustomed to seeing infants hooked up to high technology equipment, it is very startling for the parents to see their child attached to a respirator, connected to monitors and tubes, or bandaged.

The staff, rather than the physician, has to justify and explain the treatment to the parents and deal with their emotional needs. The nurses generally teach, rather than counsel, the parents about the medical care and the equipment that is being used. In general, the medical staff treat the parents as patients, with their disease being emotional in nature (Guillemin & Holstron, 1986).

Some parents are unwilling to put themselves and their infants through the trauma of high technology medicine. In a very personal article, a mother of a seriously ill newborn described her thoughts upon learning that her daughter, Amy, had hypoplastic left-heart syndrome, a malformation of the heart that impedes the pumping of blood (Vuillemot, 1988). The physicians told Amy's parents that Amy would need extensive surgery and that "probably" she would lead a normal life. Amy's parents agonized over what to do. They felt that they were being dominated by the advances in science and technology and asked themselves:

> Was it selfish to think of preserving our marriage, hoping for happier times with future children? Was it that we couldn't accept a child with a birth defect? Was it only our intense desire for a child that made us even *consider* surgery? What was best for Amy? (Vuillemot, 1988, p.100).

Amy died shortly after the parents decided not to permit the surgery.

THE COSTS

Neonatal intensive care is the most costly type of service that hospitals provide (U.S. Congress, 1987). There has been much discussion over the benefits of spending large amounts of money to save infants when the outcome is uncertain and when many of them are unlikely to lead fully productive lives (Chance, 1988; Kuhse, MacKenzie, & Singer, 1988). While several of the issues relating to the costs of neonatal intensive care are presented here, a discussion of the impact of these costs on society can be found in Chapter 5.

An important study was conducted in Hamilton-Wentworth County, Ontario of all live births between 1964 and 1969, before a neonatal intensive care program was introduced, and of all live births between 1973 and 1976, after a neonatal intensive care program was started.

One of the conclusions was that neonatal intensive care was much more cost effective for infants who weighed between 1,000 and 1,499 grams, than for infants who weighed between 500 and 999 grams. While this study was based on information from the late 1960s and mid 1970s, costs have steadily increased since then and neonatal intensive care has become much more expensive (Boyle, Torrance, Sinclair, & Horwood, 1983). Technology, too, has improved greatly. It has become very expensive to save gravely ill newborns whose outcomes and productive values are questionable. Chance (1988) remarked:

The care of severely ill infants often requires extensive use of such life-support systems as mechanically assisted ventilation and total parenteral nutrition. Surgical interventions such as ductal ligation, placement of central venous catheters and segmental bowel resection are also sometimes necessary. Although neonatal care is widely recognized to have saved many lives it is unquestionably one of modern medicine's expensive programs (p.944).

In a study reported in 1982, of 10 infants who were in a neonatal intensive care unit, Kaufman and Shepard found that the costs decreased the longer the infant remained in the neonatal intensive care unit. This was probably because the infants who survived tended to gain weight and grow stronger, thus requiring less intervention. They found that even for one fifth of the babies who had some type of disability or those who would require additional medical attention, the cost of care was economical when viewed over the lifespan of the children. They concluded that the cost of saving an infant through intensive care "is only one tenth to one twentieth the potential value society attaches to that life" (Kaufman & Shepard, 1982, p.177).

The Office of Technology Assessment (U.S. Congress, 1987), in a comprehensive report on the costs and effectiveness of neonatal intensive care units, concluded that while neonatal intensive care is very expensive the results of studies on cost effectiveness should not be used to make ethical decisions about which babies should be given treatment and which should not:

Thus, neonatal intensive care results in both increased survival and increased costs. Moreover, neonatal intensive care becomes more expensive as it is employed in increasingly marginal cases. The worth of a life saved, however, is ultimately a value judgment involving ethical and social considerations. The results from cost-effectiveness studies alone cannot guide decisions regarding who should receive care (p.7).

One of the more disturbing conclusions in the Office of Technology Assessment's report (U.S. Congress, 1987) was that the survival of low birthweight babies depends on where the baby is born. Premature and low birthweight babies tend to have a higher survival rate when they are treated in Level III hospitals:

It does appear, however, that some high-risk mothers and infants are not transferred to Level III hospitals for financial reasons. It also appears that some Level II hospitals are not appropriately transferring high-risk women and newborns because of a desire to offer competitively a full array of services even when those services do not meet the needs of patients. And most importantly, surveys show that many obstetricians and pediatricians do not have a good understanding of the prognosis for extremely low birthweight infants; they substantially underestimate the potential for survival and normal outcome (U.S. Congress, 1987, p.8).

While we can marvel at the development of high technology medicine and the life-saving care that it brings to critically ill newborns, we must also question why unequal care is provided to critically newborns. Is there one standard of care for infants who are disabled and another for infants who are not? Are the attitudes of society toward persons with disabilities reflected in the amount and type of care that is provided to newborns with disabilities? Is society willing to spend more money on a child who is not disabled than on one who is?

REFERENCES

Anspach, R.R. (1989). Life-and-death decisions and the sociology of knowledge: The case of neonatal intensive care. In L. M. Whiteford & M. L. Poland (Eds.), *New approaches to human reproduction* (pp.53-69). Boulder: Westview Press.

Boyle, M. H., Torrance, G. W., Sinclair, J., & Horwood, S. P. (1983). Economic evaluation of neonatal intensive care of very low birthweight infants. *The New England Journal of Medicine, 308,* 1330-1337.

Chance, G.W. (1988). Neonatal intensive care and cost effectiveness. *Canadian Medical Association Journal, 139,* 943-946.

Frohock, F. M. (1986). *Special care.* Chicago: University of Chicago Press.

Guillemin, J. H., & Holmstrom, L. L. (1986). *Mixed Blessings.* New York: Oxford University Press.

Gustaitis, R. & Young, E.W.D. (1986). *A Time to be Born, A Time to Die.* Reading, MA: Addison Wesley.

House, M.B.L., & Dombkiewicz, M. M. (1981). Patient care in the ICU. In G. B. Avery (Ed.)., *Neonatology: Pathophysiology and Management of the Newborn.* Philadelphia: Lippincott.

Kaufman, S. L., & Shepard, D. S. (1982). Costs of neonatal intensive care by day of stay. *Inquiry, 19,* 167-178.

Klein, N., Hack, M., Gallagher, J., & Fanaroff, A. A. (1985). Preschool performance of children with normal intelligence who were very low-birth-weight infants. *Pediatrics, 75,* 531-537.

Kuhse, H., MacKenzie, J., & Singer, P. (1988). Allocating resources in perinatal medicine: A proposal. *Australian Pediatric Journal, 24,* 235-239.

Lipsky, L. (1984). Psychosocial aspects of pediatric intensive care. In D. L. Levin, F. C. Morriss, & G. C. Moore (Eds.), *A practical guide to pediatric intensive care* (pp.449-451). St. Louis: Mosby.

McCormick, M. C. (1985). The contribution of low birth weight to infant mortality and childhood morbidity. *The New England Journal of Medicine, 312,* 82-90.

Strong, C. (1983). The tiniest newborns. *The Hastings Center Report, 13,* 14-19.

U.S. Commission on Civil Rights (1989). *Medical discrimination against children with disabilities.* Washington, DC: U.S. Commission on Civil Rights.

U. S. Congress, Office of Technology Assessment (1987). *Neonatal intensive care for low birthweight infants: Costs and effectiveness* (Health Technology Case Study 38). Washington, DC: U.S. Congress, Office of Technology Assessment.

Vuillemot, L. (1988, September 25). The fate of baby Amy. *The New York Times Magazine,* pp.38-39, 96-101.

Weir, R. (1984). *Selective nontreatment of handicapped newborns: Moral dilemmas in neonatal medicine.* New York: Oxford University Press.

Weise, R. D. (1981). Moral and ethical concerns of nurses in neonatal intensive care units. In G. B. Avery (Ed.), *Neonatology* (pp.52-53). Philadelphia: Lippincott.

Chapter 7

Family
Perspectives

The arrival of a wanted child, who is in some way disabled, elicits a multitude of feelings and a painful paradox for the parents. The pregnancy is a symbol of growth and positive familial future; the arrival of the handicapped newborn often erroneously signals "failure," the demise of family "normalcy," and perceived long term suffering and hardship for family members (Rue, 1985, p.202).

The birth of a child is usually an eagerly anticipated event. Parents are excited and have expectations about what the child will look like, who the child will resemble, and what the child's personality will be. The birth of a child with a disability can shatter these dreams and can leave the parents feeling shocked, bereaved, guilty, bitter, angry, and ashamed (Russell, 1980).

PARENTAL RESPONSIBILITIES

An assumption that is found in some studies of families with a child who has a disability is that the birth of the child brings additional burdens and responsibilities for parents and family members. While parents of children with disabilities face certain problems, it is unclear how these differ from the burdens and responsibilities of parents of children who do not have disabilities.

Rue (1985) reported that the burdens of caring for a child with a disability include:

1. an increase in family tension and conflict
2. an increase in the number of divorces
3. behavioral problems in the siblings of the child with a handicap
4. limitations on the family's social life and travel
5. physical exhaustion and emotional strain
6. an increase in the parents' anxiety over the child's future
7. sacrifices by the parents of their own careers and additional education
8. worry over hospitalization of the child
9. financial worries
10. apprehension or guilt over institutionalization.

In a small study that consisted of 25 families who had a child with a disability and an inadequately chosen sample of 5 families who did not have a child with a disability, Darling (1979) wrote that parents take on additional roles when they become parents of a child with a disability. Parents act as entrepreneurs and "become seekers and crusaders in an attempt to *fit*, on the one hand, into the services that society *does* provide, and on the other hand, to *create* the services that society overlooks" (Darling, 1979, p.235).

Parents have a number of additional jobs to perform, which include: finding a physician; locating an appropriate school program; gaining acceptance of their child by relatives; finding babysitters; paying for expensive equipment and medical care; and, finding peace for themselves.

In a survey of two-parent families of children with disabilities, both mothers and fathers reported that they wanted more information on teaching their child, on currently available and future support services, and on reading materials about parents with similar children (Bailey & Simeonsson, 1988).

In addition to these needs, the mothers wanted information about the disabling condition, opportunities to meet with other parents of children with disabilities, additional time for themselves, and assistance in paying bills.

Parents of children with mental retardation worry about having no one to take care of their children when they die. They are concerned that their children will be dependent on them for an extended period of time and are uncertain what their children's lives will be like in the future. Support services for families are inadequate in the U.S. and the social and economic burdens of raising a child with a disability are generally not shared by persons outside of the family (Rothman, 1986).

In addition to being concerned about caring for and educating their child, parents can be distressed about the economic costs of rearing a child with a disability. In 1987, the costs of raising a non-handicapped child were estimated to be $95,933 (Marsa, 1988). But there are frequently additional costs associated with bringing up a child with a handicap, especially in medical care. Bailey and Simeonsson (1988) reported that one of the needs that mothers of infants with disabilities had was assistance in paying bills for basic expenses.

The joys and pleasures of raising a child with a disability have been described in a growing body of literature written by persons with disabilities and their parents. *After the Tears* (Simons, 1987), which contains the stories of parents who had children who were disabled, provides encouragement. *Hope for the Families* (Perske, 1981) is a similar, practically oriented book, written by parents, which offers support, suggestions, and practical advice.

For example, Perske (1981) wrote that the purpose of his book was "for families who are trying to turn a tough situation into a rich experience" (p.7). Another volume written by parents is *Journey* (Massie & Massie, 1975), which relates how Robert and Suzanne Massie initially met the news that their son had hemophilia with shock and how both they and their son were strengthened by it. *Parents Speak Out* (Turnbull & Turnbull, 1985) is a book written by parents and professionals that relates the conflicts, joys, and hardships involved in raising a child with a disability. Marsha Saxton (1988), a person with spina bifida, discussed the mistaken assumptions that society has about people with disabilities. Arguing that acceptance of all people in our society will enrich all of us, she reflected:

> The assumptions I challenge include these: that having a disabled child is wholly undesirable; that the quality of life for people with disabilities is less than that for others; that we have the means to humanly decide whether some are better off never being born (Saxton, 1988, p.218).

SORROW AND STRESS

While the mother is pregnant the family fantasizes about the "perfect" child but when an infant with a disability is born, the parents begin to mourn the loss of their perfect baby. The grief process of the parents is often profound and prolonged. Some of the reactions of mourning are physical and psychological distress, preoccupation with the features of the child, hostility, abnormal patterns of behavior, guilt about behavior or thinking prior to or during the pregnancy, and actually wishing that their child would die (Kennell & Klaus, 1971; Rue, 1985). The stages of the grief process that the parents experience after their child has been diagnosed as having a disability have been described (Fletcher, 1974; Parks, 1977). In many families having a child with a severe disability, the adjustment process begins shortly after birth because that is when the diagnosis is usually made. However, in families when the disability is not diagnosed until later, the adjustment may last longer and the parents may experience more ambiguity (Blacher, Nihira, & Meyers, 1987).

Fletcher (1974) explained that after the birth of a child with a disability families proceed through three stages. The first is rejection of the child. Next, the parents begin to come to terms with their denial and anger. Finally, there is acceptance of the child as a replacement for the "lost" child. While there is disagreement over the number of stages and when parents pass through each one, a parent of a child with mental retardation has countered:

> Professionals could help parents more—and they would be more realistic—if they discarded their ideas about stages and progress. They could then begin to understand something about the deep lasting changes that life with a retarded son or daughter brings to parents and then they could begin to see that negative feelings—the shock, the guilt and the bitterness—never disappear but stay on as part of the parents' emotional life (Searle, 1978, p.23 cited by Wikler, 1981, p.284).

Interviews of 60 families with a child who has a disability in England revealed that, although some families reacted positively, there was considerable stress in these families (Lonsdale, 1978). Some mothers developed psychiatric problems or chronic back problems after the child was born (Lonsdale, 1978). Burden (1980) felt that the birth of a child with a disability is a "critical life experience" for the mother, the effects of which will interact with the effects of other critical experiences and the mother's own personality to produce a likelihood of depression or mental breakdown" (Burden, 1980, pp.122-123).

In an analysis of the family life cycle, Turnbull, Summers, and Brotherson (1986) wrote that families of children with disabilities face a number of different stressors that emanate from normal developmental stages and transitions. For instance, several of the stressors arising from the childbearing stage include getting an accurate diagnosis, finding services, and finding meaning in the disability.

Stressors associated with adolescence include adjusting to the long-term effects of the disability and coping with isolation and rejection. Finally, stressors linked with aging, planning for the care of the child after the parents die, and assigning the responsibility for the care of the child to other family members or to an institution or agency are also of concern.

The impact of the severity of the child's disability on the family is uncertain. In a multidimensional study of stress and coping abilities of parents of children with disabilities, Frey, Greenberg, and Fewell (1989) concluded that the severity of the child's disability has a profound impact on the parents. The parents reported higher stress levels when the child's ability to communicate was low. However, the level of communication affected the psychological distress of the fathers much more than it did the mothers. The gender of the child also had a strong impact on the fathers, while the coping abilities of both of the parents were related to individual beliefs.

However, another study concluded that, although mothers of children with disabilities reported higher stress levels than mothers whose children were not disabled, the severity of the disability did not seem to alter the stress levels that were reported. Byrne and Cunningham (1985) concluded that the degree of the mother's stress "appears to be more related to subjective factors than to directly measurable features—their feelings of restriction, dissatisfaction or social isolation, the ease with which they can relate to their child and the demands their children make on them" (p.850).

Roskies (1972) found in a comprehensive study of Canadian mothers of thalidomide babies that all of the mothers were sad, anxious, and pessimistic after the birth of their babies. Several of the mothers hoped that their babies would die soon; others felt that they would always have to care for their children and that they would never be independent.

In addition, the mothers had many concerns about the growth and development of the babies. They worried whether the children would ever be happy. Mothers prayed "Lord, let him live if he'll be able to be happy, but if he won't, please let him die" (Roskies, 1972, p.196).

A different view of parental adjustment was presented by Wikler, Wasnow, and Hatfield (1981). In a study of parents of children who were disabled and a comparison group of social workers, the researchers felt that parents experienced chronic sorrow rather than a "time-bound adjustment" (p.68). The chronic sorrow which the parents felt was periodic in nature—it had peaks and valleys. The intensity of the sorrow was related to the developmental stages of the child and the coping abilities of the family.

Research conducted by Beckman and Pokorni (1988) tended to support this view. In a study of 44 families of premature infants, the researchers found that the levels of stress varied with the age of the child and with the problems the family faced. These researchers reinforced the position that families are complex systems and that the dynamics of family relationships occur within this system.

In a review of the literature on sources of stress in families with a child who has mental retardation, Wikler et al. (1981) wrote that families face two types of stresses: those that are related to the difficulties associated with mental retardation (e.g., stigmatization, extended care); and those that are related to being the parent of a child with mental retardation (e.g., confusion over child care, parental grieving). Although the stresses occur throughout the lifetime of the child with mental retardation, they increase periodically when there is a discrepancy between the parents' expectations of parenting and the actual raising of a child who has mental retardation.

The anger, hopelessness, and rejection that parents experience was described in a study of families in California and Denmark who had a child with a disability. Waisbren (1980) found that parents of very young children with disabilities expressed ambivalence, sadness, disappointment, and low self-esteem. Although some parents responded positively when asked about their child, other parents viewed themselves negatively and expressed more negative feelings than families who did not have a child with a disability.

Much of the research on family stress has been conducted with mothers. It seems that parental age, socioeconomic status, and family size do not affect the amount of stress, but that the amount of stress was greater in single-parent homes than when both parents were present.

In a review of the literature, Byrne and Cunningham (1985) found that families experienced a good deal of stress upon the birth of a child with a disability, but that several variables including "the presence of multiple stresses, the life-cycle stage of the family, the family's interpretation of their situation and the integration of the family prior to the birth of the child appear to predict which families will experience stress and anxiety" (p.852).

What are the effects of parental stress on parenting? Crnic, Friedrich, and Greenberg (1983) found that stress and coping ability were related to the emotional functioning of the parents. Parents of children with mental retardation were at high risk of developing emotional and personality problems. These authors pointed out, however, that there is a need to investigate the effects of stress, coping ability, and family ecological variables on family outcomes.

It should be cautioned that the literature is conflicting about the psychological impact of a child with a disability on the family (Guess et al., 1984).

While some of the literature stresses the negative aspects, other literature emphasizes that family characteristics and family interactions before the birth of the child influence how the family responds to the child after birth. The impact of the child with a disability on the family is still under debate (Guess et al., 1984).

While many research studies and numerous reviews of the literature have been conducted on the sorrow and the stress of parents of children with disabilities, the results are equivocal. One bias found in the early literature, which may influence the design of future research studies and the delivery of services, is that children with disabilities are a burden on their families and that all families respond in a dysfunctional manner when there is a child with a disability. Only recently have studies incorporated research on family systems. It is hypothesized that many variables, both inside and outside the family, impact on and react to how families respond to having a child with a handicap. Turnbull, Summers, and Brotherson (1986) suggested that additional investigations be conducted that consider: the collaboration of researchers, practitioners, and consumers in the development of research questions and in the dissemination of the results; the use of control groups of families with nondisabled children in order to better account for the effect of the handicap on family functioning; emphasizing family strengths rather than weaknesses; and the implementation of longitudinal studies in order to examine the long-term effects of interventions.

There is still a great deal that we do not know about the sorrow and stress that parents undergo after the birth of a child with a disability. No firm conclusions can be drawn about the length of the grieving period after the birth of a child with a disability and the variables that lengthen or shorten it.

While some writers have discussed enduring sorrow, others have focused on the immediate grief that occurs when the diagnosis is made. In addition, unreplicated studies have been accepted as conclusive and there seems to be a bias that emphasizes the negative effects of having a child with a disability (Glidden, 1986).

Additional research is needed on the sources of stress and the coping abilities of the parents. It is difficult to conclude that a child with a disability makes a specific impact on the functioning of the family, that the severity of the disability increases the stress, or that families with a child with a disability function differently than families that do not have a child with a disability. As more research is conducted with better samples and control groups, the impact of a child with a disability will be more easily determined.

MOTHERS AND FATHERS

Most of the research that has been conducted on parents of children with disabilities has been conducted only with mothers. In addition, the research that has been undertaken on fathers has been only on fathers of children who have mental retardation (Lamb, 1983). Because of the scarcity of the studies that had been conducted and their ambiguousness, it is difficult to draw definite conclusions about the reactions of fathers to having a child with a disability (Byrne & Cunningham, 1985). Bristol and Gallagher (1986) emphasized that "so little is presently known regarding fathers of developmentally disabled children that information at all levels is needed" (p.95).

Why has not more research been conducted with fathers of children with disabilities? Problems associated with obtaining access to fathers as participants in research studies include:

> an absence of research paradigms that consider a triadic system rather than a dyadic one; the focus on the outcomes of intervention measures instead of research on other variables; and biases that emphasized the importance of mothers in the development of children (Bristol & Gallagher, 1986).

However, from the studies that have been conducted, several conclusions can be drawn about fathers of children with disabilities. They play two important roles (Bristol & Gallagher, 1986). The first is to provide support to the mother and the second is to convey to the family that their care for the child who is disabled is worthwhile. But there is little known about fathers' reactions to the birth of a child with a disability. It does seem that fathers tend to reject their child and to withdraw from the family. This rejection can effect the emotional development of the child, the stability of the marriage, and the emotional stability of the mother (Lamb, 1983).

Just as there are a variety of fathers, the fathers of children with mental disabilities respond in different ways to their children. While it may be difficult to distinguish between the reaction of disappointment and the stresses and strains of daily living, some fathers may be drawn closer to their children while others may pull away. McConachie (1982) speculated that "worry about the future may spur the father into teaching the child, and into battling for better services; on the other hand, it may set him apart from the mother and the child by concentrating on working harder outside the home" (pp.168-169).

Research on bonding and attachment shows that early physical contact of mothers with their babies is important to bonding. In a normal birth, the bonding and attachment process begins. The amount of time a mother spends with her newborn infant directly influences later maternal involvement. Early and long-term separation of the mother and baby may lead to a poor mother/child relationship (Lozoff, Brittenham, Trause, Kennell, & Klaus, 1977).

While the research is somewhat inconclusive (Holmes, Reich, & Pasternak, 1984), there is some evidence to suggest that when the infant and mother are separated at birth under stressful circumstances and for a prolonged period of time, the bonding may be delayed. The mother has been denied the weeks or months of emotional and physical preparation for the infant and grieves for the loss of the "normal" child (Kennell & Klaus, 1971; Lancaster, 1981).

Kennell and Klaus (1971) suggested that prolonged early separation at birth may lead to child abuse and that close emotional ties may never be developed.

However, in a study of mothers' attitudes toward preterm and term infants, researchers found that, while the birth of a preterm infant does not lead to an impaired mother/child relationship, there are two very critical periods when the mother is very anxious. The first period occurs right after the birth of the preterm infant and the second occurs when the infant is taken home from the hospital.

When the baby is first taken home, the mother is concerned about how to hold such a small child, how to care for the child's medical needs, and how to handle any feeding problems (Bidder, Crowe, & Gray, 1974). Because of the equivocal nature of the results of the research on the long-term effects of separation of high risk newborns from their mothers, additional studies are needed before firm conclusions can be drawn.

Roskies (1972), in her book *Abnormality and Normality,* interviewed 20 Canadian mothers of thalidomide babies and gathered extensive information about the mother/child relationship. During their pregnancies, several of the mothers had some insight into the possibility that their children would be born with some type of disorder. But it was not until after the delivery that the mothers were told that their children had disabilities. While the way in which each mother was told about the disability varied, Roskies found that there was a general pattern.

The mother would wake up in the delivery room and notice that the physician and nurses were acting strangely. She was told to rest and that the baby was fine. The mother was not allowed to see the baby for the first day. Various excuses were given, such as hospital policies or that the baby was weak and needed to be in an incubator. The nurses and visitors would look sad. The mother would be asked about any hereditary diseases in the family and about any medications that she had taken during the pregnancy. At last, the doctor, husband, or priest would come, draw the hospital curtain around her or take her into a separate room, and tell her. Roskies concluded that the hospital staff was anxious and ambiguous in the way they approached the mother.

The actual mothering of the child did not take place immediately. Some mothers were able to mother and care for the baby shortly after birth; other mothers felt that it took them a year or more to be able to love and care about their child.

Roskies wrote that the development of the mother/child relationship occurred in three phases. In the first stage, the mother was mourning the birth of the child and was attempting to come to terms with it. During the second stage, although the mother had many anxieties, she began to care physically for the child. By the third stage, the mother started to realize that the relationship with her child would be fulfilling, but probably not perfect.

Once the mother began to care for the child, her relationship with the child took on an intensity. This seemed to occur because the mothers were unsure whether other family members or other caretakers would adequately care for the baby. "It would appear, then, that the deformities of the child could have a bi-modal effect: initially a period of separation, but, once the mother did assume charge, a more exclusive contact with the baby than was usual" (Roskies, 1972, p.194).

In a study of mothers of children with mental retardation and mothers of children who were not mentally retarded, Watson and Midlarsky (1979) concluded that the mothers of children with retardation were overprotective. These mothers felt that the community members were more likely to have a negative opinion about children with mental retardation. Because of these beliefs, the mothers of the children with mental retardation were less likely to work full time and were more likely to use relatives to babysit rather than a neighbor.

The feeling of shame can affect the relationship between the mother and the child. In a study of mothers of European and Middle Eastern backgrounds, Margalit (1979) found that mothers with Eastern backgrounds more frequently expressed a feeling of shame.

Both maternal and paternal grandmothers have been found to be a strong source of support (Farber, 1970; Gath, 1978; Waisbren, 1980). Maternal grandmothers have provided a variety of support, including emotional support, babysitting, financial help, and gifts. Some grandmothers were left to bring up the child after the parents' marriage broke up (Gath, 1978). Farber (1970) found that the emotional support of the maternal grandmother contributed to the strength of the marriage. The support of the fraternal grandmother was reported to be of the most help by fathers (Waisbren, 1980).

Few research studies have observed the interactions between parents and their children with disabilities within the family situation. In a review of the research on parent/child interactions, Crnic, Friedrich, and Greenberg (1983) concluded that there seems to be:

> real differences in parent/retarded child involvement, affection, responsiveness, and reciprocity. Sample sizes have mostly been too small to permit generalization; and fathers, sibling, or triadic interactions have been generally ignored. Further the settings and conditions under which interactions have been observed are few. Basic descriptive research on interactions among family members is needed before more than tentative conclusions can be reached (p.132).

As with much of the literature on families, a great deal of the research on parents, children with disabilities, and their siblings is equivocal because it suffers from methodological problems—either the absence of control groups or poorly designed control groups, inadequate samples, and weak instruments.

MARITAL RELATIONSHIPS

Farber (1970), in a seminal work originally published in 1959, surveyed 240 families who had a child with severe mental retardation. Although there was no control group and despite the fact that this study was originally published in 1959, it is frequently cited in the research literature. Farber found that marital integration decreased in families with a child who has severe retardation but that the quality of the marital relationship was affected more by the marital integration before the birth of the child. As the child with the disability grew older, there was an increased likelihood of marital problems. Boys with handicaps had a greater impact on marital disruption than did girls with a disability. He concluded that the need for support services will be greater in families of children with severe mental retardation.

On the whole, marriages that are shaky to begin with seem to be worse after the birth of a child with a disability. Parents who had unhappy marriages were more likely to hide the child or to want to move to a different neighborhood. However, some marriages are strengthened after the birth of the child with the disability (Gath, 1977; 1978).

In a study that compared families who had a child with a disability with families who did not have a child with a disability, fathers felt that the child with a disability exerted a negative influence on the marriage. But, in those families in which the parents expressed positive feelings toward the child, there was more physical evidence of stress and there were negative views about the marriage (Waisbren, 1980).

Does severity of disability affect marital adjustment? Blacher, Nihira, and Meyers (1987) interviewed parents of three groups of children with mental retardation: educable mental retardation, trainable mental retardation, and severe mental retardation. No group of parents of nondisabled children was included. The authors concluded that the adjustment of families of children who were severely retarded was affected more than in the other families but that these families also reported more involvement with their children. This conclusion may reflect the greater need for involvement in families when a child is severely disabled.

There seems to be an increase in the divorce rate and the suicide rate in families with a child with a disability, but it may be difficult to determine the impact a child with a disability has on the divorce rate because there is such a high rate of divorce in our society. Carefully conducted studies with well defined samples, must be undertaken before firm conclusions can be drawn (Price-Bonham & Addison, 1978; Roesel & Lawlis, 1983).

While the research on marital relationships is conflicting, it seems that variables other than having a child with a disability influence the relationship. These other variables include the degree of disability, age and gender of the child, ability of the parents to cope, community support systems, and other ecological variables (Crnic, Friedrich, & Greenberg, 1983).

SIBLINGS

Studies of siblings of children with disabilities have also been inconclusive.

The impact of a child with a disability on siblings can be negative, positive or neutral. The adjustment of normal siblings does not seem to be affected by the gender of the child with the disability or by the family's social status.

However, Farber (1970) found that siblings were affected by the degree of dependence of the child with the disability. Sisters seemed to be held responsible for much of the care of the child with the disability.

There is some research that demonstrates that siblings of children with disabilities, especially females, may develop behavioral problems (Crnic, Friedrich, & Greenberg, 1983). A younger child with a disability seemed to affect the siblings more than an older child. Parental feelings toward the child with the disability seemed to be the strongest factor in how the siblings reacted to the child with the disability (Grossman, 1972).

Gath (1978) found that there was no discernable effect of a child with a disability on the siblings. Teacher ratings of the siblings indicated that there was no effect on the school behavior of the siblings. In addition, there was no significant difference between parental ratings of siblings in families with and without children with disabilities.

In a study of adult siblings, Zetlin (1986) found that the involvement of siblings was dependent on the individual circumstances of the siblings. The life cycle, age, marital status, geography, and parental desires and expectations helped to determine the relationships of adult siblings. Reciprocity was important to the sibling with the disability. Although not always equal in the offerings, these siblings would collect packets of jam, babysit, or purchase birthday and holiday gifts.

Nondisabled siblings can have positive relationships with their sister or brother who is disabled (Simeonsson & Bailey, 1986). Siblings can develop self-esteem and competence when they take on the role of teacher or trainer. This finding must be examined cautiously, given the results of some studies that indicate that siblings frequently take on additional care-giving roles.

Dyson, Edgar, and Crnic (1989) studied the psychological predictors of self-concept, behavior, and social competence of siblings of children who were disabled and who were not disabled. They found that children with disabilities influenced the psychological development of their siblings in a different way than did siblings of children who are not disabled.

Self-concept, behavior problems, adjustment, and social competence are all affected in siblings of children with disabilities, but for siblings who do not have a disabled brother or sister, only social competence is affected. The effect on the siblings is influenced by the attitudes of the parents, the parent's attention to personal growth, and a nurturing family environment.

Research on siblings has been equivocal and sparse. In addition, much of the research has been limited because it has been conducted with families in which the child was mentally retarded (Seligman, 1983). While some studies have shown that siblings have been harmed by the presence of a brother or sister with a disability, other research has found that the siblings have benefited. Additional research must be conducted on the emotional development of the siblings, their relationships in the community, and their mediating responses (Crnic, Friedrich, & Greenberg, 1983).

ADOPTED CHILDREN WITH DISABILITIES

In the U.S. in 1986, approximately 36,000 children with special needs who were adoptable were in foster care (Gibbs, 1989). During that year, 13,500 of these children were adopted, but more than 9,000 families adopted children from outside the U.S. and more than 25,000 adopted healthy white American infants. Thousands of children who are disabled and who are eligible for adoption remain waiting (Gibbs, 1989).

Although there is a scarcity of research on the adoption of children with disabilities, an important study was conducted in California of children with a medical condition who were adopted between 1950 and 1960 (Franklin & Massarik, 1969a, b, c). A medical condition was defined "as one requiring more than routine casework and medical consideration for placement and planning" (Franklin & Massarik, 1969a, p.461).

For most children and their families, the medical condition was not viewed as stressful, but for children with serious medical problems emotional difficulties developed. On the whole, however, Franklin and Massarik found that children with mild to severe medical problems could be successfully adopted (1969c). This study also found, like succeeding ones, that support and guidance must be provided to adoptive parents and that there must be flexibility in making adoption placements.

Nelson (1985) conducted a study of 177 families who had adopted 257 children with disabilities, most frequently behavioral or emotional in nature. Although many of the problems of the children did not disappear after they were adopted, most of the children flourished. For most families who adopted a child with special needs, the experience was successful. There were a few families in which the adoption was a negative experience. Several families dissolved the adoptions. The author felt that there was a stable pool of potentially adoptive parents, although this pool was far short of the number of families needed to adopt children with special needs.

In a follow-up study of 31 families who had adopted children, Glidden and Pursley (1989) found that in most families there was a positive adjustment to the adoption of a child with mental retardation. The mothers felt that the adoptions had worked out better than they had expected and that there had been more benefits than problems. The authors speculated that the preparation of the family prior to the adoption and the support the family receives after the child enters the home have helped the adoptions to succeed. In addition, the fact that families *chose* to adopt a child with a disability also contributes to a successful outcome.

A related study (Kadushin, 1970) of older children who had been neglected and/or abused and who were adopted after the rights of their natural parents had been terminated showed that older children who had lived under stressful conditions were able to be successfully adopted. The adoptive parents reported that they were very satisfied with their decisions to adopt older children. Many of the children developed into happy, well-adjusted people.

In a review of the literature, Glidden (1986) concluded that families who adopt children with disabilities have some knowledge about the disability, are less educated than other families who adopt, have experience in raising children, and desire to adopt a child with a disability.

Children with disabilities can bring much happiness to their adoptive families. In a study of 43 British families who had adopted 57 children with mental retardation, Glidden, Valliere, and Herbert (1988), found that the adopted children had positive effects on their families. A majority of the mothers felt that, as a result of the adoptions, they had become more tolerant, less selfish, more sympathetic and compassionate.

Why are adoptive families successful in raising a child with a disability? The families themselves may be unique, and they may be unusually strong, committed, and accepting. The adoptive family, unlike the birth family, has chosen to have a child with a disability. While the birth family may have a variety of responses, the adoptive family has planned for and is eager to welcome the child (Glidden, Valliere, & Herbert, 1988).

It is evident that additional research is needed in this area. Glidden (1986) suggested that studies include a control group of families of biological children who are disabled as well as longitudinal studies that examine families over a long period of time. In addition, other variables that affect the family must be investigated, including the degree of disability, age and gender of the child, and community support systems.

FUTURE STUDIES

Although there are obstacles to interpreting the research on families, several themes emerge. Some families do experience hardship, stress, and sorrow when a child with a disability is born. The depth and duration of their feelings depend on many variables, including the severity of the disability, marital stability, family size, economic well-being, coping ability, and the support system that is available.

For certain families, a child with a disability can bring much pleasure. Anecdotal reports by parents portray the hardships as well as the joys of raising a child with a disability. But despite methodological problems, researchers have been much more negative about the impact of a child with a disability on the family. Siblings are affected by the addition of a child with a disability and their response is related to many other variables. Adoptive families seem to manage well. This is probably because they have made a conscious decision to adopt a child with a disability and have given much thought to their decision. But for the most part, the research that has been conducted on families with a child with a disability is fragmented, inconclusive, and incomplete.

Because of methodological problems and the negative bias of some researchers, it is difficult to draw firm conclusions. In general, much of the research on the functioning of family members in families in which there is a child with a disability is equivocal and should be viewed cautiously.

Some of the research has not considered socioeconomic status, family size, the age of the child with the disability or the type and severity of the disability. Lack of control groups, the use of multiple research methods, and the lack of longitudinal studies also contribute to the inadequate research base. Researchers must better describe the sample as well as the comparison group. Strict matching procedures should be used. Statistical procedures, such as analyses of covariance, rather than t-tests, can be helpful in equating groups (Stoneman, 1989).

Besides suffering from poor research designs, there seems to be a bias toward expecting pathological functioning among the parents and siblings. The assumption that children with disabilities produce dysfunction in families should be challenged. We may find that families with children with disabilities are not much different from families whose children are not handicapped.

Outdated paradigms and theoretical research should be discarded. Research design must be linked to theory. Researchers must be aware of a bias toward looking for pathological functioning. A systems approach to the family and the family's relationship to the community and to support services should be considered.

Virtually no research has considered single-parent families, high-risk families, or how mothers and fathers who abuse drugs and alcohol react and respond to a child with a disability. Finally, while studies have searched for problems in the functioning of families, the impact of discriminatory attitudes toward persons with disabilities on families should be examined. Perhaps the problems do not reside within families but in society's attitudes toward persons with disabilities.

REFERENCES

Bailey, D. B., & Simeonsson, R. J. (1988). Assessing needs of families with handicapped infants. *The Journal of Special Education, 22,* 117-127.

Beckman, P. J., & Pokorni, J. L. (1988). A longitudinal study of families of preterm infants: Changes in stress and support over the first two years. *The Journal of Special Education, 22,* 55-65.

Bidder, R. T., Crowe, E. A., & Gray, O. P. (1974). Mothers' attitudes to preterm infants. *Archives of Disease in Childhood, 49,* 766-770.

Blacher, J., Nihira, K., & Meyers, C. E. (1987). Characteristics of home environment of families with mentally retarded children: Comparison across levels of retardation. *American Journal of Mental Deficiency, 91,* 313-320.

Bristol, M. M., & Gallahger, J. J. (1986). Research on fathers of young handicapped children. In J. J. Gallagher & P. M. Vietze (Eds.), *Families of handicapped persons* (pp.81-100). Baltimore: Paul H. Brookes.

Burden, R. L. (1980). Measuring the effects of stress on the mothers of handicapped infants: Must depression always follow? *Child: Care, Health and Development, 6,* 111-125.

Byrne, E. A., & Cunningham, C.C. (1985). The effects of mentally handicapped children on families—A conceptual review. *Journal of Child Psychiatry, 26,* 847-864.

Crnic, K. A., Friedrich, W. N., Greenberg, M. T. (1983). Adaptation of families with mentally retarded children: A model of stress, coping, and family ecology. *American Journal of Mental Deficiency, 88,* 125-138.

Darling, L. (1979). *Families against society.* Beverly Hills: Sage.

Dyson, L., Edgar, E., & Crnic, K. (1989). Psychological predictors of adjustment by siblings of developmentally disabled children. *American Journal on Mental Retardation, 94,* 292-302.

Farber, B. (1970). Effects of a severely mentally retarded child on family integration. *Monographs of the Society for Research in Child Development, 24,* (Serial No. 71). New York: Kraus Reprint Co. (Original work published in 1959).

Fletcher, J. (1974). Attitudes toward defective newborns. *The Hastings Center Studies, 2,* 21-32.

Franklin, D. S., & Massarik, F. (1969a). The adoption of children with medical conditions: Part I—Process and outcome. *Child Welfare, 48,* 459-467.

Franklin, D. S., & Massarik, F. (1969b). The adoption of children with medical conditions: Part II—The families today. *Child Welfare, 48,* 533-539.

Franklin, D. S., & Massarik, F. (1969c). The adoption of children with medical conditions: Part III—Discussions and conclusions. *Child Welfare, 48,* 595-601.

Frey, K. S., Greenberg, M. T., & Fewell, R. R. (1989). Stress and coping among parents of handicapped children: A multidimensional approach. *American Journal on Mental Retardation, 94,* 240-249.

Gath, A. (1977). The impact of an abnormal child upon the parents. *British Journal of Psychiatry, 130,* 405-410.

Gath, A. (1978). *Down's syndrome and the family.* London: Academic Press.

Gibbs, N. (1989, October 9). The baby chase. *Time, 134* (15), 86-89.

Glidden, L. M. (1986). Families who adopt mentally retarded children. In J. J. Gallagher & P. M. Vietze (Eds.), *Families of handicapped persons* (pp.129-142). Baltimore: Paul H. Brookes.

Glidden, L. M., & Pursley, J. T. (1989). Longitudinal comparisons of families who have adopted children with mental retardation. *American Journal on Mental Retardation, 94,* 272-277.

Glidden, L. M., Valliere, V. N., & Herbert, S. L. (1988). Adopted children with mental retardation: Positive family impact. *Mental Retardation, 26,* 119-125.

Grossman, F. K. (1972). *Brothers and sisters of retarded children: An exploratory study.* Syracuse: Syracuse University Press.

Guess, D., Dussault, B., Brown, F., Mulligan, M., Orelove, F., Comegys, A., & Rues, J. (1984). *Legal, Economic, Psychological, and Moral Considerations on the Practice of Withholding Medical Treatment from Infants with Congenital Defects.* Seattle: The Association for Persons with Severe Handicaps.

Holmes, D. L., Reich, J. N., & Pasternak, J. F. (1984). *The development of infants born at risk.* Hillsdale, NJ: Erlbaum.

Kadushin, A. (1970). *Adopting older children.* New York: Columbia University Press.

Kennell, J. H., & Klaus, M. H. (1971). Care of the mother of the high-risk infant. *Clinical Obstetrics and Gynecology, 14,* 926-954.

Lamb, M. E. (1983). Fathers of exceptional children. In M. Seligman (Ed.), *The family with a handicapped child* (pp.125-146). Orlando: Grune & Stratton.

Lancaster, J. (1981). Impact of intensive care on the parent-infant relationship. In S.B. Korones & J. Lancaster (Eds.), *High-risk newborn infants* (pp.354-365). St. Louis: Mosby.

Lonsdale, G. (1978). Family life with a handicapped child: The parents speak. *Child: Care, Health and Development, 4,* 99-120.

Lozoff, B, Brittenham, G. M., Trause, M. A., Kennell, J. H., & Klaus, M. H. (1977). The mother-newborn relationship: Limits of adaptability. *The Journal of Pediatrics, 91,* 1-12.

Margalit, M. (1979). Ethnic differences in expressions of shame feeling by mothers of severely handicapped children. *International Journal of Social Psychiatry, 25,* 79-81.

Marsa, L. (1988). Preparing for the costs of raising children. *Black Enterprise, 19,* 35.

Massie, R., & Massie, S. (1975). *Journey.* New York: Alfred P. Knopf.

McConachie, H. (1982). Fathers of mentally handicapped children. In N. Beail & J. McGuire (Eds.), *Fathers* (pp.144-171). London: Junction Books.

Nelson, K. A. (1985). *On the frontier of adoption: A study of special-needs adoptive families.* New York: Child Welfare League of America, Inc.

Parks, R. M. (1977). Parental reactions to the birth of a handicapped child. *Health and Social Work, 2,* 51-66.

Perske, R. (1981). *Hope for the families.* Nashville: Abington.

Price-Bonham, S., & Addison, S. (1978). Families and mentally retarded children: Emphasis on the father. *Family Coordinator, 27,* 221-230.

Roesel, R., & Lawlis, G. F. (1983). Divorce in families of genetically handicapped/mentally retarded individuals. *The American Journal of Family Therapy, 11,* 45-50.

Roskies, E. (1972). *Abnormality and normality.* Ithaca: Cornell University Press.

Rothman, B. K. (1986). *The tentative pregnancy.* New York:, Viking Press.

Rue, V. M. (1985). Death by design of handicapped newborns: The family's role and response. *Issues in Law & Medicine, 1,* 201-225.

Russell, D. S. (1980). Psychological effects on the family of a mentally retarded child. ERIC Document Reproduction Service No. ED 201 061.

Saxton, M. (1988). Prenatal screening and discriminatory attitudes about disability. *Women and Health, 13,* 217-224.

Searle, S. J. (1978). Stages of parent reaction: Mainstreaming. *The Exceptional Parent, 8,* 23-27.

Seligman, M. (1983). Siblings of handicapped persons. In M. Seligman (Ed.)., *The family with a handicapped child* (pp.147-174). Orlando: Grune & Stratton.

Simeonsson, R. J., & Bailey, Jr., D. B. (1986). Siblings of handicapped children. In J. J. Gallagher & P. M. Vietze (Eds.), *Families of handicapped persons* (pp.67-77). Baltimore: Paul H. Brookes.

Simons, R. (1987). *After the tears.* San Diego: Harcourt-Brace.

Stoneman, Z. (1989). Comparison groups in research on families with mentally retarded members: A methodological and conceptual review. *American Journal on Mental Retardation, 94,* 195-215.

Turnbull, A., Summers, J. A., & Brotherson, M. J. (1986). Family life cycle. In J. J. Gallagher & P. M. Vietze (Eds.), *Families of handicapped persons* (pp.45-65). Baltimore: Paul H. Brookes.

Turnbull, H. R., & Turnbull, A. P. (1985). *Parents speak out.* Columbus, OH: Merrill.

Waisbren, S. E. (1980). Parents' reactions after the birth of a developmentally disabled child. *American Journal of Mental Deficiency, 84,* 345-351.

Watson, R. L., & Midlarsky, E. (1979). Reactions of mothers with mentally retarded children: A social perspective. *Psychological Reports, 45,* 309-310.

Wikler, L. (1981). Chronic stresses of families of mentally retarded children. *Family Relations, 30,* 281-288.

Wikler, L., Wasnow, M., & Hatfield, E. (1981). Chronic sorrow revisited: Parent vs. professional depiction of the adjustment of parents of mentally retarded children. *American Journal of Orthopsychiatry, 51,* 63-70.

Zetlin, A. G. (1986). Mentally retarded adults and their siblings. *American Journal of Mental Deficiency, 91,* 217-225.

Chapter 8

Should Newborns with Severe Disabilities be Organ and Tissue Donors?

Medical technology has made great advances in the last few years with respect to pediatric organ transplantation. Development of medications that suppress the rejection of transplanted tissues and the improvement of surgical techniques have helped to advance progress in transplanting organs (Capron, 1987). Patients who receive kidney, heart, and liver transplants have high survival rates (Evans, 1985), but the technological gains have also raised a number of perplexing questions.

One of the most pressing problems with respect to transplantation of organs is the shortage of donor organs. For older patients who are in need of an organ donation, donations come from individuals who are usually victims of motor vehicle accidents (Capron, 1987). However, there is a severe shortage of child donors because very few infants and young children die in accidents.

It has been estimated that there is a need for approximately 400 to 500 infant hearts and kidneys and 500 to 1,000 infant livers each year (Capron, 1987). Only 40-70 % of children under the age of two who need organs receive them (Blakeslee, 1987).

DETERMINATION OF DEATH

A report issued by a Presidential Commission (1981), *Defining Death*, examined the ethical and legal issues regarding the determination of death. Because the use of respirators and other life support techniques can restore breathing, heartbeat, and blood circulation, the cessation of these functions is no longer a definitive criterion when declaring a patient dead.

Medical technology can now detect and restore brain function in some critically ill patients. The President's Commission concluded that new standards were needed to determine when death occurs and that these new standards should include "proof of an irreversible absence of functions in the entire brain, including the brain stem" (p.2). The Commission (1981) recommended that the following statute be passed by every state:

An individual who has sustained either (1) irreversible cessation of circulatory and respiratory functions, or (2) irreversible cessation of all functions of the entire brain, including the brain stem, is dead. A determination of death must be made in accordance with accepted medical standards (p.2).

To date, this statute, usually referred to as the Uniform Determination of Death Act (UDDA), while not adopted by all 50 states, has been approved by the majority of them.

Not until the last page of its report and only briefly did the President's Commission mention the determination of death in infants and children; infants with severe disabilities whose deaths were almost certain to occur were not addressed. The Commission wrote:

> The brains of infants and young children have increased resistance to damage and may recover substantial functions even after exhibiting unresponsiveness on neurological examination for longer periods than do adults. Physicians should be particularly cautious in applying neurologic criteria to determine death in children younger than five years (President's Commission, 1981, p. 166).

As of this writing, a uniform policy of determination of death among infants with severe disabilities who are critically ill does not exist.

UNIFORM ANATOMICAL
GIFT ACT

The Uniform Anatomical Gift Act (UAGA) of 1968 legalized the use of donor cards, living wills, and the right of relatives to authorize the donation of a loved one's organs (Caplan, 1983). The UAGA has been passed by all 50 states and the majority of Americans have been found to be in favor of organ transplantation and are aware of the benefits that are derived from transplantation (Stuart, Veith, & Cranford, 1981).

Although more and more states are requiring hospitals to request organ donations from relatives of patients who are dying or who have died, (Malcolm, 1986), there is a continuing shortage of infant organs. When this act was formulated, the donation of organs by infants with severe disabilities had not even been considered.

Unless patients are diagnosed as brain dead, it is considered immoral and illegal to remove organs ("Debate Raised," 1987). With the development and implementation of more intensive organ procurement procedures and the development of a national computer registry, the supply of donor organs may increase somewhat. Nevertheless, it seems that for many children who are waiting or who will be waiting for organ transplants, their needs will be unmet and these children will die waiting.

In order to avoid any conflict between health care professionals who declare an individual dead, The Hastings Center (1987) recommended that the health care provider who declares an individual to be dead not be a member of the organ transplant team and not be related to the patient.

ANENCEPHALY

Anencephaly is an irreversible congenital disorder in which the cerebral cortices, the centers of higher cognitive operations, are missing. It is one of the neural tube defects. Many infants born with this disorder are stillborn because their brains lack the structures necessary to maintain life (Barowsky, 1987). It has been estimated that approximately 2,000 to 3,000 babies who are anencephalic are born each year (Capron, 1987).

Under current laws, organ donors must be brain dead. This means that the patient's other bodily functions, such as heartbeat and elimination, are still functioning with the support of machines. Using these criteria, not all infants with anencephaly can be diagnosed as brain dead. There has been considerable debate about whether to include infants who have anencephaly in the standards of the UDDA.

Capron (1987) wrote that one of the reasons why infants with anencephaly should not be included under the UDDA is because physicians view these infants as dying, but not dead. Capron (1987) pointed out that although the majority of these infants die within the first few days of birth, a small number will survive at least to the seventh day after birth. Several infants who were diagnosed as having anencephaly had been misdiagnosed, and have survived.

The organs of babies with anencephaly usually atrophy as the baby slowly dies, making the babies ineligible to be organ donors when they do die. Organ transplant centers have rejected these babies as organ donors because they have not been considered dead under current laws and medical standards (Blakeslee, 1987). If a respirator is used to keep the infant alive, it may be difficult to determine when death occurs.

ORGAN DONATION

In an attempt to help parents come to terms with anencephaly and to meet the shortage of donor organs, the donation of organs from newborns with anencephaly has been considered and, in several cases, undertaken. Five German doctors (Holzgreve, Beller, Buchholz, Hansmann, & Kohler, 1987) have reported the successful transplantation of three kidneys from two infants with anencephaly.

The first infant was delivered at 38 weeks of gestation, after the parents had been informed about the diagnosis of anencephaly. At birth, the infant's blood pressure was maintained and the child was given ventilatory support for 45 minutes after the delivery until surgery was performed and the kidneys were removed.

The second case was a twin whose sibling was healthy. In this instance, the infants were delivered by Cesarean section at 36 weeks of gestation. The twin with anencephaly was kept alive for approximately 60 minutes until the kidneys were removed. In both cases, the physicians reported that the parents "expressed relief of their suffering and mourning when the option of donating the kidneys of their infants became available to them" (Holzgreve et al., 1987, pp.1069-1070).

In the first case known in the United States, a baby with anencephaly donated her heart to another infant. The donor, named Baby Gabrielle, was born in Canada and flown to California where her heart was given to an infant boy who was born just a few hours before the surgery.

Baby Gabrielle was placed on a respirator and kept alive until it was determined that she would be unable to survive without the assistance of the respirator. At that time, it was determined that Baby Gabrielle met the legal criteria for brain death. The physicians determined that brain death occurred when Baby Gabrielle did not breathe on her own when the respirator was turned off for three minutes.

Since her organs were healthy, the heart transplant surgery could be undertaken. One of the physicians, reported that, "The parents insisted that they wanted their infant's organs used. They wanted to see that their baby would touch others and contribute to life in some way" (Blakeslee, 1987, p.A18).

As of this writing, there are no actively functioning transplantation programs for the use of organs from infants with anencephaly (Truog & Fletcher, 1989).

FAMILY PERSPECTIVES

There is some evidence that suggests that donor families believe that the donation of a loved one's organs is "the highest form of charity" (Bartucci & Seller, 1986, p.401). Bartucci and Seller (1986) contacted 23 donor families who had received thank-you letters for donating the organs of their loved ones. Although it is unknown if any of the respondents were parents of children with a disabling condition, 89% of the families felt that organ donation helped to ease their grief and 84% of the families reported that they did not have any regrets about organ donation.

Not all of the families were positive about the donation process, however. Several expressed the need for more communication with the transplant team about the transplantation process and which organs would be transplanted. Two families grieved that their loved one had to be maintained on a respirator and undergo surgery after dying in order to make the transplant possible. One mother regretted that although she had wanted to donate her child's liver, a recipient could not be located in time.

Donation of a close relative's organs can ease the grief and the knowledge that part of your loved one continues to survive can be comforting. In one case, upon learning that their first child would be born with anencephaly, a couple chose to continue with the pregnancy so that the infant's organs could be donated. They pleaded with hospital administrators and legislators to allow medical personnel to keep their infant alive long enough so that the infant's organs could be transplanted.

The mother, Brenda Winner, is quoted as saying, "When we found out about the baby, that was devastating enough, but when we discovered that the organs would all be healthy and normal and that babies who need a liver or heart couldn't get them, well, that's when we started getting into it" ("Debate Raised," 1987, p.A23). But the baby was stillborn, leaving most of the infant's organs useless for transplantation.

The donation of a loved one's organs can be very stressful to family members. Besides suffering the loss of a loved one, who may have died tragically, the donor may not appear to be dead. Machines are still connected to the body and these keep the organs alive. Monitoring of body functions continues. The body is warm, has good color, and the chest may be moving up and down as the ventilator keeps the body breathing. One child poignantly expressed the conflict felt by the family, " 'That's my brother,' said the little boy, 'He's dead and they're taking him to surgery' " (Youngner et al., 1985, p.322).

Gold, Kirkpatrick, Fricker, and Zitelli (1986) analyzed the stages of the transplantation process as described by a group of parents of children who were waiting for organ transplants. Although the medical prognosis and care varies for every child and for the type of transplant, the authors believed that "the families appear to face identical emotional stresses and use similar coping mechanisms" (Gold et al., 1986, p.739).

These authors divided the transplantation process that parents face into three stages: preoperative psychosocial issues, perioperative psychosocial issues, and long-term psychosocial issues. Each stage includes a number of substages. In the preoperative stage, while the child is waiting for a transplant, the parents are busy making arrangements and caring for their child. Although parents work to prevent their child from becoming sicker, only the children who are critically ill receive transplants. During this stage, parents feel guilty:

> One mother described her guilt: 'I find it very difficult to pray for the life of my child at the expense of another.' Parents have talked about an approaching holiday and the increased number of donor organs it will bring from the high rate of automobile accidents (Gold et al., 1986, p.740).

Once a donor is located and the child is prepared for surgery, the parents begin the perioperative stage. During surgery the parents reported that they felt numb and anxious. After the surgery, still fearful, some families inquired about the sex and age of the donor and how the donor died. Around the second and third weeks after the transplant, the process of integrating the organ begins:

> Families work toward integrating the new organ in a number of ways. For example, questioning the medical staff about the donor's age, sex, and circumstances of death helps the parents accept the reality of the new organ.

As the patient progresses and is able to express feelings once again, the parents' fantasies and fears are lessened (Gold et al., 1986, p.741).

During the perioperative stage, fears about rejection and infection begin to increase. Although the child can feel well one day, complications can arise unexpectedly and the child's health can vary from day to day. Parents feel powerless and anxious about their child. If a child dies, all of the parents suffer. As the child recovers, parents become more confident and emotionally stable.

During the third stage, the long-term postoperative stage, the biggest fear of the parents is that the donor organ will be rejected. Parents may be overprotective of the child and unnecessarily set restrictions on the child's activities. Once the child is home, the mother's role and activities change. Used to caring for a critically ill child, the mother must make a major adjustment. One mother was quoted as saying, "I'm so afraid that I don't know who I am. I feel like I've lost my identity" (Gold et al., 1986, p.742). During this adjustment process, parents worry about the future for their child. Medical expenses, side-effects of the medications, and whether their child will be able to have children are some of the anxieties that these parents have.

Gold et al. (1986) concluded:

Advances in medical technology that make transplantation possible also exacerbate the ethical dilemma that the physician faces in caring for the dying child. The decision between transplantation and allowing a child to die has never been more difficult. This fact becomes even more poignant when considering the mother's comment that her child "only traded one disease for another disease" (p.743).

CARE GIVERS' PERSPECTIVES

The maintenance of newborns with anencephaly on life support machines until the removal of organs can take place raises troubling issues for medical personnel. Although potential donors have irreversibly lost brain function, they may not appear to be dead. Because the body is maintained by medical technology, it feels warm and has color.

Health professionals are required to monitor the "dead" person's bodily functions. Because of this, health care providers may experience some ambivalence and confusion "about having to perform cardiopulmonary resuscitation on a patient who has been declared dead, whereas a 'do not resuscitate' order has been written for a living patient in the next bed (Youngner et al., 1985, p.321).

When the organ donor is taken to the operating room where the organs are removed, the body does not appear dead. Taking it to the operating room, where the usual procedure is to save lives, causes emotional discomfort for family members and health care workers. This is accentuated when the removal procedure is finished, the machines are disconnected and the body is transported to the morgue (Youngner et al., 1985).

The donation of the organs of infants with anencephaly raises troubling questions for medical personnel:

> First of all, although medical and surgical interventions are sometimes painful, invasive, and even disfiguring (e.g., amputation of limbs), they are justified as being necessary to the achievement of the primary goal—the patient's welfare. During retrieval, the donor's welfare no longer provides the rationale for these aggressive procedures. Secondly, the organ recovery process seems to violate a more general respect for persons, which obligates us to treat human beings as ends in themselves rather than mere means to other ends. Thirdly, organ retrieval may be viewed as being disrespectful to the dead. Our cultural and moral traditions demand that we respect not only recently dead bodies but also graves that are centuries old (Youngner et al., 1985, p.322).

Harrison (1986) presented a fictional case in which a pregnant woman and her husband were told that their child had been diagnosed as having anencephaly. While the parents and physicians agreed that the organs of their child should be donated, many moral and ethical questions for medical personnel were raised:

> If they (medical personnel) accepted the mother's wish to have the baby be an organ donor, were they under an obligation to try to resuscitate the infant if it was stillborn? What steps should they take to try and support the child considering that babies born with this condition normally received no aggressive treatment in the nursery? Perhaps most confusing was the question of when death should and could be pronounced (Harrison, 1986, p.21).

In an attempt to alleviate the discomfort of medical personnel and family members, Youngner et al. (1985) recommended that the following alternatives be considered: educational and emotional support be provided to the health care workers; family members be allowed to see their loved one after the removal of the organs and after the machines and tubes have been disconnected; and the adoption of a moment of silence by medical personnel after the infant has been disconnected from the life support machines.

WHO GETS ON THE
WAITING LIST?

When the Loma Linda Medical Center in California placed a newborn with anencephaly on a respirator for the first time for the purpose of transplanting the infant's organs in February 1988, the question of who and how children get placed on the waiting list for organs was raised (Blakeslee, 1988).

Because there are far more children in need of organ transplants than the number of organs available, a critical question is: "who gets on the waiting list?" Because transplants are based on the ability to pay, children whose families are poor or uninsured are not put on national waiting lists. Transplants are viewed as experimental by state and federal medical insurance programs, so these funds are not available to help pay for the costs of the transplant procedure.

ETHICAL PERSPECTIVES

When anencephaly and other severe handicaps are diagnosed *in utero*, parents are faced with an agonizing dilemma. If the pregnancy is carried to term, their child will be stillborn or face almost certain death within a few days or months of birth.

An alternative that is usually presented to parents of babies with anencephaly is selective abortion. Selective abortion is the termination of a fetus following positive identification of fetal defects. Another alternative would be to carry the fetus with anencephaly to term with the intention of donating the baby's organs once it was born.

Harrison (1986) suggested the development of a new term to refer to anencephalic newborns. Rather than using the term "brain dead," which does not cover all anencephalic newborns, he suggested the use of the term "brain absent." Harrison (1986) argued that this term would be more appropriate because some anencephalic children are born with a brain stem that does function for hours, and in some cases, days. If the brain stem is functioning, the organs cannot be removed. During this time the organs are deteriorating and they will not be usable when the child is considered brain dead.

The adoption of the term "brain absent" would allow the use of these organs. This term would apply only to newborns with anencephaly and not to other newborns who are severely disabled. Under these conditions, the removal of the organs should take place quickly. The gestation period should not be prolonged and the use of life support machines would be considered inappropriate.

Decisions concerning the termination of pregnancy and evaluations to determine brain absence should be conducted by a team of professionals not involved with the transplant. In all cases, parents should be prohibited from making any financial gains by permitting their infant to be an organ donor (Holzgreve et al., 1987).

The "brain absent" approach can be likened to inserting a wedge into a slippery slope (Mahowald, Silver & Ratcheson, 1987). While fetuses or newborns with disabilities less devastating are protected, newborns with anencephaly are not. By permitting the donation of organs from one infant with one type of severe handicapping condition, will we be opening the dam to permit organ donation from infants with other types of severe handicaps?

Still another recommendation has been to consider infants with anencephaly as being without "personhood." Harrison (1986) argued against this recommendation, writing, "it is difficult to reach a consensus about the personhood and what constitutes humanness...this approach raises a specter of abuse in which other fetuses or newborns, possibly with less severe disabilities, might be denied personhood" (p.22).

Truog and Fletcher (1989) proposed a new standard for determining death—one that would permit the donation of organs from infants with anencephaly:

> People are dead if they have a distinct and precisely definable condition characterized by the absence of integrative brain function, such that somatic death is uniformly imminent (p.389).

According to Truog and Fletcher (1989), there are only two types of persons that meet this standard—people who are brain dead and infants with anencephaly. Underlying this proposal is the assertion that infants with anencephaly are not alive and thus, retrieving their organs is acceptable.

Parents would be able to donate the infant's organs shortly after the diagnosis of anencephaly is made, thus avoiding the critical problem of the deterioration of the organs during the dying process. Truog and Fletcher (1989) recommended that the Uniform Anatomical Gift Act be amended to include their proposal.

Medical research conducted with newborns with anencephaly tends to support the conclusion that current laws are inadequate to ensure the successful transplantation of organs from infants with anencephaly (Peabody, Emery, & Ashwai, 1989).

With the consent of their families, the care of 12 infants with anencephaly was changed for one week. Six infants received intensive care from birth and six infants were kept comfortable and received intensive care only when death seemed imminent. For those infants receiving intensive care, only 1 met the criteria for brain death during the week. Of the infants who received a delay in intensive care, the organs were not appropriate for donation.

The authors concluded that "it is not feasible, within the restrictions imposed by current requirements of total brain death, to procure from anencephalic infants a substantial number of hearts and livers for transplantation" (Peabody, Emery, Ashwai, 1989, p. 350). From this study, it seems that modifications in existing laws and policies will have to be made, before extensive use of infants with anencephaly as organ donors can occur.

There have been several attempts to legalize the donation of organs by newborns with anencephaly (Capron, 1987). The first, a proposal submitted to the California Senate, would have allowed a change in the Uniform Determination of Death Act that would have permitted the donation of organs from infants with anencephaly. This proposal was withdrawn. The second proposal was a bill submitted to the New Jersey Assembly that would allow the donation of organs of a newborn with anencephaly and permit an exception to the Uniform Anatomical Gift Act. Capron (1987) wrote that "Both of these attempts are well-meaning but in my view misguided. They would create very substantial problems, as well as undermine the very goal they seek" (p.6).

Capron suggested that "medical ingenuity should be directed toward finding ways to care for dying anencephalic (and other) babies so that when they become brain-dead, they can be organ donors (with their parents' permission)" (1987, p.9). Society should not pursue a course of abandoning living newborns for the purpose of transplanting organs.

Arguing in favor of the rights of persons with severe neurological disabilities, Coulter (1988) wrote that removing the organs from an infant who is not brain dead is a form of active euthanasia and constitutes direct medical killing of the infant:

> Those who seek to permit this active euthanasia must recognize the significant ethical, legal, and historical risks inherent in such a policy. On the other hand, those whose concern for safeguarding the rights of persons with severe disabilities leads them to oppose active euthanasia must acknowledge the suffering of infants who might benefit from organ transplantation as well as their families. Perhaps some way can be found to provide organs without the necessity of active euthanasia (p.74).

The American Association on Mental Retardation (AAMR) has opposed the donation of organs from infants who have not been diagnosed as brain dead. In 1988, the following resolution was adopted by the AAMR Board of Directors:

RESOLUTION ON ORGAN TRANSPLANTATION

WHEREAS, Recent attempts to transplant organs from infants born with anencephaly to mentally typical infants in need of healthy organs have highlighted the risks faced by infants, children, and adults with disabilities that their lives will be devalued and that they will be forced to sacrifice their own lives in order to donate organs to people without disabilities.

HERETOFORE, be it resolved that the American Association on Mental Retardation reaffirms its Resolution on Infants with Handicaps and further urges: Organ donation should only occur when the donor is brain-dead and where proper consent has been obtained. Brain death is defined as the absence of all brain activity including brain stem reflexes (for example, the proposed donor cannot breathe on his or her own). Neither anencephaly nor any other disability alone meets the strict criteria of brain death. The determination of brain death should be made by physicians who are not on the transplant team in order to minimize the possibility of conflict of interest or the appearance of conflict of interest. People with mental retardation should be accorded the same consideration as other individuals when considered for organ transplants ("BOD passes," 1988, p.4).

TRANSPLANTATION OF FETAL
TISSUE

Compounding the debate, the transplantation of fetal tissue to patients with Parkinson's disease, Alzheimer's disease, diabetes, and other disorders has received a great deal of attention. Although controversial, there is some evidence that supports the transplantation of fetal tissue in the alleviation of these conditions.

Fetal brain tissue can grow considerably in size in an adult brain and different types of fetal tissue can be transplanted to other brains. In addition, the site of implantation and exact tissue match may not be critical to the success of the implantation.

Although preliminary results look promising, this research is viewed with a great deal of caution. Edwin Kiester, quoting one researcher, wrote that research must discover "how to keep more tissue alive and to find ways to make the cells grow greater distances and make proper connections with the proper areas. In the end the goal has to be to achieve profound behavioral change every time we perform the procedure" (Kiester, 1986, p.38).

Physicians in Mexico have been transplanting tissue from the brains and from the adrenal glands of spontaneously aborted fetuses to adults who suffered from Parkinson's disease for several years (Rohter, 1988).

In Mexico, there are many more restrictions on abortion than there are in the U. S. Abortions can only be performed for "therapeutic" reasons, which are "cases of rape and instances in which a mother's life is in danger or she is determined to be suffering from diseases that could affect the fetus, such as measles or AIDS" (Rohter, 1988, p.B13).

Dr. Madrazo, the developer of this transplant procedure, explained the steps he followed to assure that consent was obtained for the removal of the fetal brain tissue. Only the tissue of spontaneously aborted fetuses was used; tissue from fetuses who were electively aborted was not used. Although consent only had to be obtained from the mother, he also obtained the consent of the father. The death of the fetus was pronounced by two physicians who were not part of the transplant team. The patients who were to be the recipients of the fetal transplant were aware that they could not undergo surgery until a fetus was available.

A number of ethical dilemmas have been raised regarding the use of fetal tissue in brain transplants (Mahowald et al., 1987; Rohter, 1988). Mahowald said:

> By proceeding the way they have, the Mexicans appear to be speaking to the very grave concerns that have been raised about separating the procedure by which the tissue is made available from that through which it is used, as well as questions about informed consent and the exploitation of women (Rohter, 1988, p.B13).

The Mexican physicians decided to use spontaneously aborted fetuses in order to avoid the concerns of anti-abortion and religious groups, who feared that some fetuses may be purposely conceived and then aborted so that family members of the mothers could be aided. But the practice of using spontaneously aborted fetuses has also been questioned because these fetuses may have brain tissue that is abnormal (Rohter, 1988).

Mahowald et al. (1987) suggested that certain moral requirements be adhered to when transplanting fetal tissue:

> consent of proxy; a significant research or therapeutic goal, and ascertainment that other (less problematic) means of obtaining the goal are not available (p.12).

Mahowald et al. (1987) also raised the issue of whether tissue should be taken from nonviable fetuses. While there is much controversy on this issue, they wrote that it is morally defensible to take tissue from nonviable living fetuses if dead fetuses are unavailable or are unsuitable donors. This proposal could, if carried out, be applied to fetuses with anencephaly and other severe handicaps. Parents of these fetuses might be encouraged to undergo selective abortion so that the fetus could be a tissue donor.

In 1989, the American Medical Association (AMA) issued a report (Bohigian & Patterson, 1989) that reviewed the research on transplantation of fetal tissue. The report stated that the transplantation of fetal tissue is permitted and that transplantation is covered by the legal requirements of the Uniform Anatomical Gift Act.

According to this report, transplantation of fetal tissue is permitted if physicians follow ethical guidelines for transplantation and when:

- Fetal tissue is not provided in exchange for financial remuneration above that which is necessary to cover reasonable expenses.
- The recipient of the tissue is not designated by the donor.
- A final decision regarding abortion is made before initiating discussion of the transplantation use of fetal tissue.
- Decisions regarding the technique used to induce abortion, as well as the timing of the abortion in relation to gestational age of the fetus, are based on concern for the safety of the pregnant woman.
- Health care personnel involved in the termination of a particular pregnancy do not participate in or receive any benefit from the transplantation of tissue from the abortus of the same pregnancy.
- Informed consent on behalf of both the donor and the recipient is obtained in accordance with applicable law (Bohigian & Patterson, 1989, p.11).

In the United States, the U. S. government has banned the use of fetal brain tissue from fetuses that have been deliberately aborted (Wheeler, 1988), but still permits the use of spontaneously aborted fetuses as tissue donors.

As of this writing, the U. S. government has not developed federal guidelines for the transplantation of fetal tissue (Wheeler, 1988).

WHAT NEXT?

New developments in both organ and tissue donation occur almost daily. As we progress, it is hoped that some of these dilemmas will be resolved. Care and compassion must be extended to those who require organ and tissue donations, but, as advocates for persons with disabilities, many of whom are unable to advocate for themselves, we must take heed of the direction the American Association on Mental Retardation has recommended:

People with mental retardation should be accorded the same consideration as other individuals when considered for organ donation ("BOD passes," 1988, p.4).

REFERENCES

Barowsky, E. I. (1987). Anencephaly. In C. R. Reynolds & L. Mann (Eds.), *Encyclopedia of Special Education*, Vol. 1, (p.91), New York: John Wiley & Sons.

Bartucci, M. R., & Seller, M. C. (1986). Donor family responses to kidney recipient letters of thanks. *Transplantation Proceedings, 18,* 401-405.

Blakeslee, S. (1987, October 19). Baby born without brain kept alive to give heart. *The New York Times,* pp.1, B9.

Blakeslee, S. (1988, February 23). Quandries of timing on infant organs. *The New York Times,* p.C2.

BOD passes resolutions on AIDS and transplants. (1988, July). *News & Notes-Quarterly Newsletter of the American Association on Mental Retardation.* p.4.

Bohigian, G. M., & Patterson, R. H. (1989). *Medical Applications of Fetal Tissue Transplantation.* Joint Report of the Council on Scientific Affairs and The Council on Ethical and Judicial Affairs. Available from the American Medical Association, Chicago, IL.

Caplan, A. L. (1983). Organ transplants: The costs of success. *The Hastings Center Report, 13,* 23-32.

Capron, A. M. (1987). Anencephalic donors: Separate the dead from the dying. *The Hastings Center Report, 17,* p.5-8.

Coulter, D. L. (1988). Beyond baby Doe: Does infant transplantation justify euthanasia? *Journal of the Association for Persons with Severe Handicaps, 13,* 71-75.

Debate raised over doomed fetus's organs. (1987, December 7). *The New York Times,* p.A23.

Evans, R. W. (1985). The socioeconomics of organ transplantation. *Transplantation Proceedings, 17*(6), 129-136.

Gold, L. M., Kirkpatrick, B. S., Fricker, F. J., & Zitelli, B. J. (1986). Psychosocial issues in pediatric organ transplantation: The parents' perspective. *Pediatrics, 77*(5), 738-744.

Harrison, M. R. (1986). The anencephalic newborn as organ donor. *The Hastings Center Report, 16* (2), 21-22.

The Hastings Center (1987). *Guidelines on the Termination of Life-Sustaining Treatment and the Care of the Dying.* Bloomington: Indiana University Press.

Holzgreve, W., Beller, F., Buchholz, B., Hansmann, M., & Kohler, K. (1987). Kidney transplantation from anencephalic donors. *Medical Intelligence, 316,* 1069-1070.

Kiester, E. (1986). Spare parts for damaged brains. *Science, 231,* 33-38.

Malcolm, A. H. (1986, June 1). Human-organ transplants gain with new state laws. *The New York Times,* pp.1, 28.

Mahowald, M., Silver, J., & Ratcheson, R. A. (1987). The ethical options in transplanting fetal tissue. *The Hastings Center Report, 17* (1), pp.9-15.

Peabody, J. L., Emery, J. R., & Ashwai, S. (1989). Experience with anencephalic infants as prospective organ donors. *The New England Journal of Medicine, 321*, 344-350.

President's Commission (1981). *Defining Death.* Washington, DC: U. S. Government Printing Office.

Rohter, L. (1988, Jan. 7). Implanted fetal tissue aids Parkinson's patients. *The New York Times*, p.B13.

Stuart, F. P., Veith, F. J., & Cranford, R. E. (1981). Brain death laws and patterns of consent to remove organs for transplantation from cadavers in the United States and 28 other countries. *Transplantation, 31* (4), 238-244.

Truog, R. D., & Fletcher, J. C. (1989). Can organs be transplanted before brain death? *The New England Journal of Medicine, 321*, 388-393.

Wheeler, D. L. (1988, April 27). Transplanting fetal cells from elective abortions banned in NIH studies. *The Chronicle of Higher Education*, pp.A5, A12.

Youngner, A. M., Bartlett, E. T., Cascorbi, H. F., Hau, T., Jackson, D.L., Mahowald, M. B., & Martin, B. J. (1985). Psychosocial and ethical implications of organ donors. *The New England Journal of Medicine, 313*(5), 321-323.

Chapter 9   # Through the Looking Glass

...as we seek wisdom in the use of our human-made tools, reaching beyond what is given, we must always be keenly aware of our inescapable frailties...especially those that arise—not from any defect in our genes—but from a failure in our vision (Nolan & Swenson, 1988, p.46).

The lightning advance of technology in the diagnosis of fetal defects, the management and treatment of the fetus *in utero* and in the neonatal intensive care unit have a number of implications for imperiled infants, their families, medical care personnel, and society. Morality and technology do interact (Fletcher, 1983).

Public policy develops as a result of the interaction between ethical beliefs and technological progress. Developments in technology are progressing at a rapid pace. Before we can understand and fully use new technologies, newer experimental technologies are developed. Fueled by developments in technology, profound issues have been raised about the effects of technology on the fetus, on the infant, and on society.

MAPPING THE GENES

In January 1989, the Human Genome Project was formally started (Jaroff, 1989). The goal of the project is to map the human genome. A genome provides the blueprint for human development. Approximately 100,000 genes occupy a genome. About 4,550 have been identified. One of the most important benefits of this project will be to discover which genes are responsible for various diseases and birth defects.

The discovery of which genes are responsible for specific conditions will dramatically change the way medical care is delivered. Already, with the identification of genes for Tay-Sachs disease, Huntington's disease, cystic fibrosis, and sickle-cell anemia, the emphasis is on the prevention of the disease. Prevention, right now, is through the conscious decision not to have children or through selective abortion.

Early identification through prenatal diagnosis will help physicians to treat more diseases *in utero*. In addition, parents can make preparations before the birth of their child for appropriate medical care and early intervention services after the child is born. Although the identification of genes has far outpaced advances in treatment, gene therapy, which is the insertion of "good" genes into a patient's cells, will be possible in the future.

ADVANCES IN DIAGNOSIS

Because of the advances in prenatal diagnosis and their widespread use, fetal abnormalities can be identified as early as the sixth week of pregnancy. Early diagnosis allows the parents and the physician to treat the fetus, if treatment is a possibility, make any special preparations for the birth, or to selectively abort the fetus. Each of these alternatives can decrease medical and psychological risks.

Neuroimaging techniques provide information on body function and an understanding of treatment (Stark, Menolascino, & Goldsbury, 1988). But progress in diagnostic technologies has outpaced the advances in treatment, giving rise to a new dilemma: when and for whom and at what cost should diagnostic technologies be used when treatment may be uncertain or unknown?

Some fetuses can be treated *in utero*. When treatment is a possibility, which fetuses should be treated and which should be aborted? When treatment is not a possibility, should the pregnancy be continued? Who should make these decisions? Should the ability to pay be a consideration? What standards should be used—the mother's, the father's, the physician's, or society's?

ADVANCES IN FETAL THERAPY

Prenatal diagnostic techniques can diagnose genetic, metabolic, anatomical, and immunological disorders in the developing fetus (Callahan, 1986). Conditions for which the fetus can now be treated *in utero* include pulmonary immaturity, anemia, hypothyroidism, goiter, hydrocephalus, urethral obstruction, and diaphragmatic hernia (Harrison, Golbus, & Filly, 1981).

Treatments include giving the mother medications and nutrients, injecting medication and nutrients into the fetus, and surgery on the fetus (which also necessitates surgery on the mother) (Harrison et al., 1981).

Although treatment of the fetus can be an alternative to selective abortion, it seems apparent that the fetus, whose rights are uncertain, is being increasingly viewed as a "patient" (Callahan, 1986). Harrison, Golbus, and Filly (1981) wrote that because fetal disorders can be detected and in some cases treated, "the fetus with a treatable birth defect is on the threshold of becoming a patient" (p.777).

So, while there seems to be a "patient," whether the patient should have any rights and which rights should be granted are unclear. What about the rights of the mother? If the fetus is viewed as a "patient," the rights of the fetus and the mother may be seen as competing with each other.

While these issues are being debated on the larger political scene, there are legal questions with which the Congress, state legislatures, and the courts will be confronted. Besides the legal implications, there are psychological ones as well (Callahan, 1986). Harrison et al. (1981) raised some of these questions:

> Who makes decisions for the fetus? How can the risk of intervention be weighed against the burden of the malformation itself? (p.777)

Courts in Georgia and Colorado have already had to confront the issue of fetal rights. Judges in these states ordered that Cesarean sections be performed on women in order to save the lives of their fetuses (Callahan, 1986). In each of these cases, the rights of the mother were overruled. A California court prosecuted a woman, whose son was born brain dead because of amphetamines in his body, for abusing her fetus ("Brain-Dead Birth," 1986).

The juxtaposition between fetal rights and women's rights also occurs in the work place. There have been concerns about pregnant women working in potentially hazardous environments and the effect of these environments on the fetuses.

For example, women working with video display terminals for long periods each day may be exposing their fetuses to potential damage. Can and should women be required to work in safe environments when they are pregnant? With what regulations should employers be forced to comply when an employee is pregnant and the health of the fetus is at stake?

The emerging rights of the fetus pose other dilemmas. At what point do the rights of the fetus outweigh those of the mother? Otten (1985) raised other questions concerning parental and fetal rights. Should a woman be forced to undergo a Cesarean section or take blood transfusions to save a fetus? Should a mother on drugs be forced to submit to tests and treatment for addiction?

Should a woman be obliged to undergo a procedure involving fetal surgery if it is required to treat a damaged fetus? After a child is born and it is exposed to hazardous conditions and substances, the mother may be accused of child abuse. Should a mother be required to avoid hazardous conditions while she is pregnant? The obligation of the woman to her fetus, with the few exceptions cited previously, has not been questioned in the courts.

What about the role of the physician? Physicians, who have a life-preserving role, may choose to save the fetus rather than to carry out the mother's wishes for an abortion. If both the mother and the fetus are viewed as patients, to which patient is the physician responsible? In difficult cases, more than one physician will probably be involved with the pregnancy: the obstetrician will care for the mother and the perinatologist will care for the fetus (Lenow, 1966). What will happen if fetal surgery is recommended and the mother refuses? The physicians may be in conflict and the issue will probably be left to the courts to decide.

When resources are scarce, questions have been raised about their distribution (Beeson, Douglas, & Lunsford, 1983). Although prenatal diagnosis is viewed as a preventive program and research has shown that prevention programs are cost effective, other prevention programs, such as prenatal care are also cost effective. To which programs should resources be channeled? Which patients should have access to prenatal diagnostic programs and who establishes the criteria for access?

NEONATAL INTENSIVE CARE

The use of high technology medical care in the neonatal intensive care unit saves the lives of infants who a few years ago would have been doomed to die. Very low birthweight babies, infants who are premature, and others that have serious medical problems now survive thanks to suction machines, respirators, transfusions, monitoring equipment, and highly technical laboratory tests.

Infants physicians once thought could not live now survive. The costs of saving these high technology babies has been and continues to be debated. Is it cost effective to spend more than $100,000 to save an infant? In a time of budget constraints, should money be used to care for these fragile infants or should it be used for other socially beneficial programs? How should these decisions be made?

While tiny, fetus-like babies struggle to survive, technology persists in producing bleeps, buzzes, hums, and blinking colored lights. Once the newborns are admitted to a neonatal intensive care unit, the technology goes into action. As an increasing number of critically ill babies survive, there are more children who are disabled (U.S. Congress, 1987).

Many of these children will require additional medical attention and support throughout their lives:

> The cost to society increases as neonatal intensive care is provided to the very lowest birthweight infants, but it would be unethical and illegal to categorically deny treatment. So far, technology cannot determine at birth which infants are doomed to severely handicapped lives. Physicians, in conjunction with parents, have traditionally grappled with decisions about treatment for premature and sick newborns—and they must continue to do this (U.S. Congress, 1987, p.7).

While the benefits, pleasures, and joys of raising a child with a disability have been described, they are not widely known. Educational programs and community support services can be very effective in helping the family and the child with a disability. Why have these benefits not been more widely publicized? Why have organizations that advocate on behalf of persons with disabilities not been more vocal about promoting the advantages and joys of raising a child with a disability?

It is not only on the societal level that these questions are raised. What about the benefits to the family? Should families take on the financial and social responsibilities of caring for a child with a disability? In the United States, which has a tradition of aggressive medical treatment, high-technology interventions are commonplace. Who decides which infants should be treated? Should it be the courts, the legislatures, the physicians, or the parents?

DISCRIMINATION AND DISABILITIES

One theme of this book has been that, almost from the beginning of history and continuing into present times, people with disabilities have been targets of discrimination. The type of discrimination has only been limited by the imagination.

Based on surveys of health care providers, the testimony of experts, investigative reporting, and journal articles, the U.S. Commission on Civil Rights (1989) concluded that there is "likelihood of widespread and continuing denials of lifesaving treatment to children with disabilities" (p.148). The statement issued by the American Association on Mental Retardation (Berkowitz, 1983), *Principles of Treatment of Disabled Infants,* firmly opposes "discrimination of any type against any individual with a disability/disabilities regardless of the nature or severity of the disability" (p.263).

The complexity of new technologies, their profound implications, and the breathtaking pace of development make it difficult for society to reach an understanding of the emerging technologies (Nolan & Swenson, 1988). A child with a disability may be discriminated against because no one got to the child "in time" to prevent the child from being born or to prevent the child from surviving.

This lack of understanding may lead to stigmatization of newly identified conditions and to continued discrimination against people with disabilities. Nolan and Swenson (1988) feared that, with identification of more and more genes, it will become increasingly difficult for society to tolerate differences. They urged:

> Perhaps we should actively encourage greater public acceptance of variation and vulnerability. We may not yet be either willing or able to adopt an ethic of genetic screening and intervention that is responsive to the desire to promote individual and societal well-being while not destructive of the richness of expression inherent in nature and human society (Nolan & Swenson, 1988, p.45).

DILEMMAS OF TECHNOLOGY

Rifkin (1983), an opponent of biotechnology, wrote that society must reevaluate its relationship with nature. He cautioned that as technology progresses, the world deteriorates. A biologically engineered world is a lonely, unfeeling, and controlling world. Now is the time to take stock before disaster strikes. The world must be preserved for future generations and we must be able to live in harmony with nature. Should we heed Rifkin's pleas?

Technology has far outpaced society's ability to cope with the ethical dilemmas it has raised. While technology and ethical standards do interact, it is evident that the development of public policy is lagging far behind the advances in technology. While technology and medical science continue to progress, decisions are being made and questions are being asked: Who should live? Who shall live? Who shall die?

REFERENCES

Beeson, D., Douglas, R., & Lunsford, T. F. (1983). Prenatal diagnosis of fetal disorders. Part II: Issues and implications. *Birth, 10,* 233-241.

Berkowitz, A. (1983). National news. *Mental Retardation, 21,* 263-264.

Brain-dead birth case tests fetal-rights law. (1986, Oct. 2). *Portland Press Herald,* p.11.

Callahan, D. (1986). How technology is reframing the abortion debate. *The Hastings Center Report, 16,* 33-42.

Fletcher, J. C. (1983). Ethics and trends in applied human genetics. *Birth Defects, 19,* 143-158.

Harrison, M., Golbus, M., & Filly, R. (1981). Management of the fetus with a correctable congential defect. *Journal of the American Medical Association, 246,* 774-777.

Jaroff, L. (1989, March 20). The gene hunt. *Time, 133*(12), 63-67.

Lenow, J. L. (1966). The fetus as a patient: Emerging rights as a person? *American Journal of Law and Medicine, 9,* 1-29.

Nolan, K., & Swenson, S. (1988). New tools, new dilemmas: Genetic frontiers. *The Hastings Center Report, 18,* 40-46.

Otten, A. (1985, April 12). Women's rights vs. fetal rights looms as thorny and divisive issue. *Wall Street Journal,* p.27.

Rifkin, J. (1983). *Algeny.* New York: Viking Press.

Stark, J. A., Menolascino, F. J., & Goldsbury, T. L. (1988). An updated search for the prevention of mental retardation. In F. J. Menolascino & J. A. Stark (Eds.), *Preventive and Curative Intervention in Mental Retardation* (pp.3-25). Baltimore: Paul H. Brookes.

U.S. Commission on Civil Rights. (1989). *Medical discrimination against children with disabilities.* Washington, DC: U.S. Commission on Civil Rights.

U.S. Congress, Office of Technology Assessment. (1987). *Neonatal intensive care for low birthweight infants: Costs and effectiveness.* Health Technology Case Study 38. Washington, DC: U.S. Congress, Office of Technology Assessment.

About the Author

Libby G. Cohen is Professor of Special Education at the University of Southern Maine. She received her Ed.D. from Boston University and is the author of articles and books about the education of children and youth with disabilities and ethical issues relating to persons with disabilities. A previous holder of the Walter E. Russell Chair in Philosophy and Education at the University of Southern Maine, she resides in Cape Elizabeth, Maine with her husband Les, and son Seth.